Capstone Coach
for Nursing
Excellence

Capstone Coach
for Nursing
Excellence

Linda Campbell
PhD, RN, CNS, CNE
Professor
Loretto Heights School of
  Nursing
Rueckert-Hartman College for
  Health Professions
Regis University
Denver, Colorado

Marcia A. Gilbert
DNP, APRN-CNP(Fam)
Associate Professor
Loretto Heights School of
  Nursing
Rueckert-Hartman College for
  Health Professions
Regis University
Denver, Colorado

Gary R. Laustsen
PhD, APRN-CNP(Fam),
FAANP, FAAN
Associate Professor
School of Nursing
Oregon Health and Science
  University
La Grande, Oregon

F.A. Davis Company • Philadelphia

F. A. Davis Company
1915 Arch Street
Philadelphia, PA 19103

Printed in the United States of America

Last digit indicates print number: 10 9 8 7 6 5 4 3 2 1

Director of Content Development: Darlene D. Pedersen
Acquisitions Editor: Thomas A. Ciavarella
Project Editor: Jamie M. Elfrank, MA
Design and Illustration Manager: Carolyn O'Brien

As new scientific information becomes available through basic and clinical research, recommended treatments and drug therapies undergo changes. The author(s) and publisher have done everything possible to make this book accurate, up to date, and in accord with accepted standards at the time of publication. The author(s), editors, and publisher are not responsible for errors or omissions or for consequences from application of the book, and make no warranty, expressed or implied, in regard to the contents of the book. Any practice described in this book should be applied by the reader in accordance with professional standards of care used in regard to the unique circumstances that may apply in each situation. The reader is advised always to check product information (package inserts) for changes and new information regarding dose and contraindications before administering any drug. Caution is especially urged when using new or infrequently ordered drugs.

Library of Congress Cataloging-in-Publication Data

Campbell, Linda (Professor of nursing), author.
  [Clinical coach for nursing excellence]
  Capstone coach for nursing excellence / Linda Campbell, Marcia A. Gilbert, Gary R. Laustsen.
— Second edition.
      p. ; cm.
  Preceded by Clinical coach for nursing excellence / Linda Campbell, Marcia A. Gilbert, Gary R. Laustsen. c2010.
  Includes bibliographical references and index.
  ISBN 978-0-8036-3907-2
  I. Gilbert, Marcia A. (Marcia Ann), author. II. Laustsen, Gary R., author. III. Title.
  [DNLM: 1. Nursing Process—United States. 2. Clinical Competence—United States.
3. Education, Nursing—United States. 4. Nurse's Role—United States. WY 100 AA1]
  RT86.7
  610.73—dc23
                                    2013037963

This second edition is dedicated once again to the nurses from our past, present, and future: shining lamps of nursing knowledge!

Preface

We three faculty members continue to draw inspiration for this second edition resource from our devotion to nursing excellence and our love of teaching today's gifted and motivated nursing students. We also endeavor to meet the needs of our profession, which is experiencing an acute shortage not only of new graduate bedside nurses but also in progressive career options, including preceptors, charge nurses, advanced practice nurses, and nursing faculty. At the same time, continued emphasis on quality patient care—termed Quality and Safety Education for Nurses (QSEN)—calls for RNs to master the knowledge, skills, and attitudes that promote desired outcomes across the continuum of health-care delivery (Disch, 2012).

Professional nursing organizations have immersed themselves in ways to balance the current nursing shortage with quality patient care. Of enduring importance, during its annual education summit in 2005, the National League for Nursing identified three critical milestones for the nursing school graduate:

- Passing the NCLEX-RN examination
- Continuing in nursing past the first 2 to 3 years
- Enjoying a lengthy career in progressive nursing roles

Capstone Coach for Nursing Excellence provides the keys to accelerate your transition from student through the first two milestones so that you may enjoy the same full and rewarding career in nursing that we have experienced. Our motto is:

"We hand you the keys. You accelerate to RN practice."

We have written this clinical guide and application manual for the following audiences:

- Senior nursing students
- Nursing interns and externs
- Newly graduated nurses in residencies and other new graduate programs
- RNs through their first 2 to 3 years of practice

Most textbooks are 3 inches thick, and we use them for learning or reference. This second edition clinical guide "cuts to the chase" to accelerate nursing students' transition to practice. Although this guide offers many features of an application manual, it is *not* an A-to-Z catch-all. Rather, it is a manual of often-used elements that many students find difficult to master. This guide directly helps you to:

- Master key concepts and skills.
- Make important connections between evidence and practice.
- Stand out to potential employers in your capstone or senior nursing practicum.
- Prepare for and pass the NCLEX-RN examination with confidence and ease.
- Flourish in your first 2 years of RN practice and beyond.

We are pleased to gather previously scattered resources into one clinical guide for you. We predict that *Capstone Coach for Nursing Excellence* will become your favorite, always-in-the-backpack resource. You will want to delve into this guide as a senior nursing student. You will dog-ear its pages as a nursing intern or extern, as a new graduate, and as an RN in your initial couple of years of practice. Designed for regular and repeated use, its features will grab your attention, promote your mastery of critical content, and help you develop problem-solving skills that distinguish you from peers. We encourage you to put your mastery to use as a servant-leader devoted to quality patient care, safety, evidence-based nursing practice, and exemplary interprofessional collaboration.

We have selected and organized content according to our experiences in nursing, education, and business. Our overarching desire, or philosophy, is to promote **professional pride**. We believe that nursing's visibility and value will follow naturally from increased pride. We use a map, Benner's 1984 theory of skill acquisition (Benner, 2001), to guide the way. Benner provides the path, and we contribute the vehicle from time-tested assertions. Some of these assertions have endured for years; others come from cutting-edge literature. All of these assertions resonate with professional pride:

- "Begin with the end in mind" (Covey, 1989, p. 95).
- Pursue consciously competent practice (Benner, 2001).
- Have the knowledge, skills, and attitudes (KSAs) necessary to improve continuously the quality and safety of the health-care systems within which you work (Cronenwett et al., 2007; Disch, 2012).
- Improve "patient care and the work environment through support of evidence-based practice" (Goode, 2000, p. 222).
- Use Servant Leadership as a structural basis for hope and healing (Greenleaf, 2002; Yancer, 2012).
- "Say *yes* to wow!" (Peters, 1999, p. 309) to accelerate reflective journaling.

We value the feedback and recommendations received about the first edition of *Clinical Coach for Nursing Excellence*. It is our great pleasure and a source of our own professional pride to incorporate updated information, emerging topics, and desired content in a second edition.

First, we revised the title of this resource to *Capstone Coach for Nursing Excellence, Second Edition*, to capture the optimal timing of its use, beginning with senior nursing students. Although a few students wished their programs required this cut-to-the-chase resource earlier or in place of more comprehensive textbooks, short-cuts typically result in gaps in knowledge, skills, or requisite attitudes. Nursing curricula are carefully crafted to meet standards for quality and safety. According to Benner (2001), "novices" must immerse themselves in sufficient depth and breadth to acquire the pattern recognition that prepares them to transition to the professional workforce as "advanced beginners." This resource is designed as a culminating guide. It may benefit students as a companion to a comprehensive textbook, but it is not a replacement.

We hope you will embrace and enjoy the journey to become a registered nurse! Picture yourself driving around a mountain toward its summit. Steep switchbacks require time and tax your engine, but you can improve your performance through an approach that honors the complexity of the profession, the skill acquisition needed to save lives and promote desired outcomes, and the components of stewardship necessary not only for today's health-care delivery systems but also for health-promoting self-care. The first time around the mountain develops a broad clinical foundation, via a fundamentals course, skills laboratories and simulations, and a beginning medical-surgical course. The second time around the mountain provides a combination of repeated and new clinical content as well as more skills laboratories and simulations via advanced medical-surgical and specialty courses. The view may be similar, but your vantage point is higher and you recognize more elements of quality and safe nursing care. The third time around the mountain continues your upward spiral via a capstone or practicum course. Confidence from ascending even higher adds depth, personally and professionally, and related patterns emerge. Powerful motivation and far-reaching dividends are now in view, arising from the correlation between doing well in your program and passing the NCLEX-RN examination the first time you take it.

Second, we retained the overall structure of 10 chapters, with no change in their titles but with updated content to reflect current best and evidence-based practice. Updates come from recent nursing literature, professional conferences, and the experience of graduates. Chief among updates are directives for increased professionalism in high-tech environments, advances in genomic health care, and expanding recognition of nurses as stewards of holistic human health and healing. RNs increasingly serve on boards, cut costs, and participate in a pharmacological trend that educates patients about "farm-acology," which is the study of nutrient-dense ways of eating as a first line of defense against disease. We also prominently display *I-SBAR-R* (Identification-Situation-Background-Assessment-Recommendation-Readback), which is the interprofessional communication strategy recommended by the QSEN Institute, and confirm findings from recent literature on readiness for practice.

Third, we heeded recommendations to pack the second edition with even more practical content. The following additions reflect our priority for need-to-know, leading-edge content:

- Decision trees for laboratory values related to changes in condition, diagnoses, medications, and procedures.
- A PEAK Performance Box about IV solutions, explaining the nurse's role in their safe administration.
- A PEAK Performance Box about anticipatory guidance for grief, including a section on hospice and palliative care from a recent graduate's volunteer experience.
- A PEAK Performance Box with the proven path to passing the NCLEX-RN examination the first time taken.
- More Coach Quadrants and Consults with explicit communication strategies and styles.
- More Coach Consults for working with diverse populations, including essential phrases in Spanish and French with referral to *Taber's Cyclopedic Medical Dictionary* for many more phrases, and ways to increase sensitivity for other cultures and sexual orientations.
- Evidence-Based Practice Boxes related to quality and safety, including early warning scores, bedside reporting, and patient identifiers.

We view our efforts as a way to express ourselves as "super-mentors." Russo (2007) describes a super-mentor as "a selfless soul who is an expert teacher, life coach and networker-extraordinaire all wrapped into one" and asserts that "becoming a super-mentor is as worthy an aspiration as, say, curing cancer, understanding an ecosystem or identifying the stuff that makes up the Universe" (p. 881). We hope to have you regard us as your super-mentors to address intensely felt difficulties in making the transition from nursing student to practicing RN. We would love to hear from you as your exciting future in nursing unfolds!

Reviewers

Carol Fanutti, EdD, MS, RN, CNE
Director of Nursing
Trocaire College
Buffalo, New York

Joanne Folstad, RN, BSN, MCEd(c)
Instructor, Nursing Education Program of Saskatchewan
Saskatchewan Institute of Applied Science and Technology, Kelsey Campus
Saskatoon, Saskatchewan
Canada

Cathy M. Ford, MS, RN, FNP-BC
Associate Degree Nursing Program Coordinator
Tri-County Technical College
Pendleton, South Carolina

Emily Harder, BScN, RN
Nursing Faculty
Saskatchewan Institute of Applied Science and Technology, Kelsey Campus
Saskatoon, Saskatchewan
Canada

Tara R. Jones, RN, MSN, ACNP-BC, PNP-BC, APRN-BC
Nursing Faculty
Central Alabama Community College
Childersburg, Alabama

Linda Krueger, RN, MSN, EdS
Nursing Instructor
Chippewa Valley Technical College
Eau Claire, Wisconsin

Mary Ann Liddy, RNC, BSN, MSN/Ed
Nursing Faculty
Clayton State University
Atlanta, Georgia

Jan Lloyd-Vossen, RN, BScN, MN
Faculty, Nursing Education Program of Saskatchewan
Saskatchewan Institute of Applied Science and Technology, Kelsey Campus
Saskatoon, Saskatchewan
Canada

Jane A. Madden, MSN, RN
Professor of Nursing
Pikes Peak Community College
Colorado Springs, Colorado

Suzanne Marnocha, RN, MSN, PhD, CCRN
Director, Traditional Undergraduate Nursing Program
University of Wisconsin Oshkosh
Oshkosh, Wisconsin

Alicia Oucharek Mattheis, RN, BScN, MN, CPN(C)
Faculty, Nursing Education Program
Saskatchewan Institute of Applied Science and Technology, Kelsey Campus
Saskatoon, Saskatchewan
Canada

Donna M. Penn, RN, MSN, CNE
Assistant Professor, Nursing
Mercer County Community College
Trenton, New Jersey

Rose M. Powell, PhD, RN
Assistant Professor
Stephen F. Austin State University
Nacogdoches, Texas

Teri-Anne Smith Schroeder, RPN, RN, ET, BScN, HCL, IIWCC, MCEd
Faculty, Nursing Education Program
Saskatchewan Institute of Applied Science and Technology, Kelsey Campus
Saskatoon, Saskatchewan
Canada

Mary Pat Szutenbach, RN, PhD
Associate Professor
Regis University
Denver, Colorado

Deonna Tanner, RN, MSN
Assistant Professor of Nursing
Clayton State University
Morrow, Georgia

Table of Contents

1 Foundations: Providing a Framework to Accelerate Your Transition to Practicing RN

Foundations: Providing a Framework to Accelerate Your Transition to Practicing RN

Welcome to *Capstone Coach for Nursing Excellence.* We wrote this clinical guide to accelerate your transition to becoming a practicing RN. In fact, if you read the preface, you know our motto: "We hand you the keys. You accelerate to RN practice."

This second-edition guide promotes consciously competent nursing practice by identifying potential difficulties for you *before* you enter the nursing workforce and elevating your confidence *after* you graduate. As you learned in nursing school, cutting-edge RN practice depends on philosophy, theory, nursing process, and best evidence. You already have the philosophy and desire to become a registered nurse; we provide a nursing theory or map by which you can track your progress "from novice to expert." We revisit the nursing process because it comprises the first six American Nurses Association (ANA) standards of professional practice. We have also researched the best evidence or practice elements that many students and newer nurses find difficult to master. Six of these difficulties are listed in Box 1–1, "Why Is *Capstone Coach for Nursing Excellence* Important?"

In this first chapter, we present foundational content designed to make clinical content in Chapters 2 through 10 more understandable and memorable. We selected this content not only from our own experiences as

---

Box 1–1 Why Is *Capstone Coach for Nursing Excellence* Important?

Casey and colleagues surveyed 270 new graduate RNs to gauge graduate nurses' experiences. Analysis of responses to open-ended questions revealed six themes, cited here in order of frequency and intensity of difficulty in making the transition from student to RN:

1. Lack of confidence in skill performance; deficits in critical thinking and clinical knowledge.
2. Relationships with peers and preceptors.
3. Struggles with dependence on others, yet wanting to be independent practitioners.
4. Frustrations with the work environment.
5. Organization and priority-setting skills.
6. Communication with physicians.

Note: These research results have held up in subsequent studies but can be mitigated by a nursing student internship or senior nursing practicum (Casey, Fink, Jaynes, Campbell, Cook, & Wilson, 2011; Steen, Gould, Raingruber, & Hill, 2011).

Adapted from Casey, Fink, Krugman, & Propst, 2004, p. 307.

---

nurses and faculty but also from contributions of high-profile leaders in nursing and business. Chief among them are:

- Patricia Benner, PhD, RN, FAAN, whose 1984 model of skill acquisition has become a well-accepted theory of nursing students' consistently observed progression "from novice to expert." In 2001, the importance of Benner's theory received additional endorsement through its republication in a 25th anniversary edition of her book. In 2011, Benner's theory garnered more commendation from online publication of the Tildens' influential book review.
- Joann Disch, PhD, RN, FAAN, Director of the Katharine J. Densford International Center for Nursing Leadership in Minneapolis, Minnesota, whose 2012 article updated the impact of "Quality and Safety Education for Nurses." Popularly known as QSEN (pronounced "kew-sen"), this rapidly accepted effort enjoys elevated status as the "QSEN Institute" and conveys much of what it means to be a capable and respected nurse. The related website (at www.qsen.org) no longer requires a

user account, making its valuable resources readily accessible to faculty, students, and practicing nurses.

- Colleen Goode, PhD, RN, FAAN, whose presentations and publications document her own evolution from research utilization to evidence-based practice (EBP) in nursing. Further credence for the essential nature of EBP comes from its inclusion as one of six QSEN competencies and its explication in dedicated textbooks.

- The late Stephen R. Covey, MBA, DRE, whose publications and presentations in principle-centered leadership have achieved international renown. His phrase, "Begin with the end in mind," will serve your entire career, and his depiction of pursuits in a quadrant model inspired our own Coach Quadrants, which are discussed later in this chapter.

- The late Robert Greenleaf, a management and education researcher, who coined the term *servant leadership* in 1969. Our service-mandated profession continues to embrace this approach, which aligns with the QSEN competency related to patient-centered care.

- James C. Collins, MBA, who with Stanford business professor Jerry I. Porras wrote *Built to Last: Successful Habits of Visionary Companies*. They coined the phrase, "Embrace the genius of the *and*," which we do throughout this guide, such as by presenting nursing *and* business tools. We explain this concept more fully in the following section titled "You and *Capstone Coach for Nursing Excellence*."

- Tom Peters, MBA, PhD, who wrote *The Circle of Innovation* and coined the phrase, "Say *yes* to WOW!" We hope you say *yes* to WOW throughout your nursing career!

You and *Capstone Coach for Nursing Excellence*

You may feel at least as nervous about launching your career in nursing as you did when you first got behind the steering wheel of a car. You may wonder how you will fare as a new graduate nurse, especially when many of your concerns appear among the daunting list of transitional difficulties presented in Box 1–1, "Why Is *Capstone Coach for Nursing Excellence* Important?" The answer is easy: immerse yourself in this guide, and consider us your personal coaches.

Coaches take pride in helping charges face reality, and wise coaches do not permit wallowing in gut-wrenching words such as *lack, deficit, struggle,* and *frustration*. Instead, you will learn to apply the "genius of the *and*," a theme that emerged from a Stanford study of outstanding businesses. The "genius of the *and*" acknowledges the reality of simultaneous driving and restraining forces. For example, improved outcomes in health-care delivery have resulted from driving forces, such as a national surge in nurse-managed clinics to increase accessibility, availability, and affordability of primary health care. At the same time, advanced practice nurses in these clinics have offered restraining forces related to overuse of the health-care system through their emphasis on anticipatory guidance, health promotion, and disease prevention strategies.

The "genius of the *and*" also honors the ability to cope with these simultaneous forces and counters a tendency to view potential outcomes as all or nothing, either/or, or only positive or only negative. In reality, you will experience frustration *and* triumph. You may focus on struggles, however, because advances occur sporadically enough that you fail to notice them. For example, you may depend on a preceptor for multistep procedures such as a central line dressing change even while you are achieving independence in equally daunting areas such as shift organization. You will notice progress more often if you consciously engage in reflective professional practice, which is the ability to look back in order to look forward with more clarity and discernment. Try these strategies:

- **Set aside time to think.** Aim for 15 to 20 minutes every day. By adding time for reflection to the usual quick thinking required in the nursing role, you may avoid the "all or nothing" trap that often accompanies more impulsive reactions. This time in reflection is particularly helpful if you catch yourself saying "yes" when you mean "no."
- **Identify three or more alternatives to a dilemma.** This strategy prevents "either/or" thinking.
- **Think more objectively about issues by setting up a pro-and-con table.** This action disrupts seeing situations as completely positive or completely negative.
- **Ask yourself questions that incorporate changes and transitions you want for the future:** "What do I know now that can help me when I get off orientation?"
- **Take pride in the active listening skills and powers of observation you are developing in your nursing role.**

The "genius of the *and*" extends to the powerful emotions you may feel as a nurse. For example, it is undeniably sad when a patient dies, and many nurses wonder how they can have pleasant emotions at the same time. In fact, nurses often grapple with extended periods of sadness, especially if they intensify sad occurrences by experiencing them as "horrible" or "devastating." We encourage you to resist such magnifications and to attempt to feel less sad until you are calm. The following actions support this mature and self-nurturing approach:

- Consider that the opposite of "sad" is *not* "happy." The opposite of "sad" is "not sad." Happiness is on a different continuum of joyful emotions. As a result, happiness can coexist with less enjoyable emotions when you appreciate the "genius of the *and*."
- Insist on debriefing with preceptors or peers after a sad outcome, as you did during nursing school classes or post-clinical conferences. Experienced nurses appear callous when they dismiss newer nurses' need to debrief a patient's death. In truth, they may have acquired the ability to feel less sad but are unable to articulate this coping mechanism. You may have to remind them of the need to process patients' deaths.
- Set a timer for 30 minutes, and allow yourself to feel sad until the buzzer sounds. Each subsequent day, set the timer for 1 minute less. As the end of 1 month approaches, most nurses have unburdened their sadness and feel calm. If this strategy does not relieve your sorrow, contact your employee assistance program for additional help.

Capstone Coach for Nursing Excellence also accelerates your transition to becoming a practicing RN through its features, such as various margin notes and clinical exemplars. In addition, PEAK Performance boxes identify relevant strategies that promote the **P**urpose, **E**vidence, **A**ction, and **K**nowledge nursing students and RNs need to achieve desired outcomes for patients. Throughout this guide, we coach in the following ways:

- Explaining concepts, roles, and actions that are difficult to master.
- Illustrating pattern recognition of "consciously competent" thoughts, words, deeds, and habits.
- Guiding your practice of critical skills.
- Inspiring you to envision yourself in safe, competent practice— well beyond your starting point as a nursing student.

Our former students tell us that a particularly helpful tip was to anticipate themselves a year into safe, competent practice while they were still students. As a result, they had the energy, will, and emotional stability needed to persevere through every milestone along the way:

- Taking final examinations.
- Preparing for and taking the NCLEX-RN licensing examination (including waiting for results).
- Seeking out and interviewing for new graduate RN positions.
- Engaging in new employee and unit orientations.

Alumni surveys revealed that our former students benefited from seeing themselves as consciously competent. They completed orientations sooner, had more respectful interactions with peers and preceptors, and advanced to float nurse and preceptor roles less than 1 year into RN practice. A favorite comment from a community agency was, "We don't interview your graduates. We hire them."

Peak Performance Key No. 1: Philosophy and Theory of RN Practice

Our first key is to explain hard-to-understand foundational concepts. We seek to increase your understanding of the underlying purpose, evidence, action, and knowledge related to RN practice. We begin by translating abstract words such as *philosophy* and *theory* into everyday language that you can remember and embrace:

- **Philosophy = Desire:** Our greatest desire for you is to take and show pride in professional nursing.
- **Theory = Map:** We use Benner's 1984 Model of Skill Acquisition (Benner, 2001), presented in PEAK Performance Key No. 2 in more detail.

Once you have a map, you can confidently select your path, which will serve as a framework for professional nursing practice. National faculty for the QSEN Institute recommends these six competencies for any path in nursing (Cronenwett et al, 2007; Disch, 2012):

1. Patient-centered care, in which the patient (or designee) is a co-partner with the health-care team.
2. Teamwork and collaboration, which takes place within nursing and interprofessional teams.
3. EBP, which integrates clinical expertise, best evidence, and patient preferences for delivery of optimal health care.
4. Quality improvement, which uses data for monitoring and continuous improvement of health-care systems.

5. Safety, which minimizes risk of harm to patients and providers.
6. Informatics, which uses information and technology in all aspects of care, including clinical decision making.

As your coaches, we add four more elements to create a comprehensive framework that supports professional nursing pride:

1. Spectral thinking, which specifies ways of thinking to obtain a more complete picture of any clinical puzzle or problem (see related PEAK Performance Box).
2. Reflective journaling, which enhances and documents your thinking and changes your role in the framework from recipient of learning to active participant.
3. Energy management, which underlies your ability to meet the demands of your framework *and* personal life.
4. Servant leadership, which promotes hope, healing, and health not only for individuals but also for organizations.

Peak Performance Key No. 2: Clinical Progression From Novice to Expert

We chose Benner's model of skill acquisition (Fig. 1–1) not only as another articulation of "begin with the end in mind" but also as a map. Its theoretical progression "from novice to expert" will help you envision and track your development in professional nursing.

▲ PEAK PERFORMANCE: SPECTRAL THINKING

International nursing leader Daniel Pesut, PhD, RN, FAAN, cites six ways of thinking. Taken together, they constitute spectral, or comprehensive, thinking and provide the foundation for clinical reasoning:

1. Critical thinking, which nursing students know well as quality of thought. The Foundation for Critical Thinking (www.criticalthinking.org) defines critical thinking with a list of universal intellectual standards: clarity, accuracy, precision, relevance, depth, breadth, logic, significance, and fairness.
2. Creative thinking, which considers alternative solutions, including the sometimes opposite point of view of other people. Nurses' inclination toward empathy facilitates the desired creativity.
3. Reflective thinking, which comes from engaging in self-talk. A mirror may promote authentic reflective thinking. When you talk to yourself in a mirror, you can catch nonverbal expressions, such as flinching, frowning,

Continued

or smiling, that will help you better analyze and evaluate something that has happened.

4. System thinking, which considers the possibility of behind-the-scenes elements or unquestioned structures. For example, you notice that patient transfers go smoothly between only one intensive care unit (ICU) and step-down unit, and you wonder why. You learn that their charge nurses meet for breakfast once a month to maintain goodwill and collaborative relationships. To accelerate your ability to acquire system thinking, challenge the unconscious reply, "Because that's how we've always done it."

5. Network thinking, which acknowledges and attempts to respond to complexity in the health-care delivery system. To enhance network thinking while beginning as a nursing student, notice situations that demand an urgent response. Note how often they occur and what resources are required to address crises.

6. Predictive thinking, which searches for patterns by using an "if/then" approach. For example, "If I ask Patient A about her pain level before taking in her scheduled medications, then I might save a trip to the Pyxis."

Novice and Advanced Beginner

According to Benner (2001), nursing students perform as novices. Two factors characterize the novice stage:

1. Dependence on rules: to counter a lack of experience.
2. Frustration: when a rule applies in one situation but not in another.

Senior nursing students must transition from novice to advanced beginner to meet universal expectations for safe practice as new graduate nurses. This stage depends on two factors:

1. Real-life clinical experiences.
2. Recognition of recurrent and meaningful patterns.

Clinical context

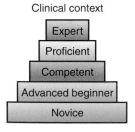

FIGURE 1–1: Benner's model of skill acquisition: from novice to expert.

You will notice achievement of this step to advanced beginner when you no longer need to ask a preceptor for "the rule" about an element of nursing practice. Instead, you will use principles to guide your actions and anticipate exceptions to rules based on unit-specific clinical experiences. For example, RNs working in a multispecialty surgical ICU had a "rule" to use soft restraints on intubated patients' wrists to prevent premature extubation. However, application of the rule had exceptions based on the principle that the use of restraints was to promote patient safety.

A woman with Marfan syndrome was one such exception. She had received a new heart valve by means of open heart surgery. She remained intubated and ventilated for several days postoperatively but was fully awake and aware. In establishing a care plan, the primary RN and patient negotiated the use of soft restraints only during sleep. When the patient was awake, her wrists remained untied to allow written communication. This 38-year-old woman had a lot to say! She wrote about her syndrome, numerous surgeries, quality of life, and hopes for the future. She filled a yellow legal pad during her stay and was grateful for RNs who not only engaged in meaningful "conversation" with her but also allowed her to express herself as fully as possible during her intubation.

To accelerate your transition from novice to advanced beginner:

- Anticipate orders based on similar assessments, and document new knowledge in your clinical log or journal.
- Discuss surprises with your preceptor.
- In your care plans, track the amount of time you spend performing interventions. For example, your confidence will soar when you can do a central line dressing change in less time. At first this sterile procedure may take 30 minutes and be accompanied by requests for someone else to bring supplies. With experience you may need only 10 minutes and no help.

> **ALERT** !
>
> Lapses in sterile technique require immediate remediation. A breach in sterile technique is a critical violation of patient safety.

In addition to developing a principle-driven approach to nursing care, advanced beginners also must demonstrate mastery of critical clinical skills. Your nursing program no doubt provided you with a multipage checklist of every conceivable psychomotor skill, which you updated during skills and simulation laboratories and clinical rotations. This kind of comprehensive checklist does not identify the "must have" skills that promote confidence in senior nursing students, their patients, and their preceptors. Box 1–2, "Essential Skills for the Generalist RN," lists essential skills and groups them according to the steps of the nursing process.

Box 1–2 Essential Skills for the Generalist RN

The following skills are grouped according to general nursing skills and the nursing process. These are considered basic skills that a generalist nurse should be comfortable performing after completing nursing school.

1. General
   - Body mechanics
   - Bed making
   - Code (COR) response
   - Collaboration with health-care team and family
   - Delegation
   - Disaster response
   - Isolation precautions
   - Nursing documentation
   - Perioperative care (preoperative/postoperative)
   - Postmortem care
   - Principles of infection control (hand washing, levels of precautions)
   - Prioritization
   - Sterile technique
2. Assessment
   - Basic "head-to-toe" physical assessment
   - Epidural assessment
   - Health history interviewing
   - Intake and output (I&O)
   - Newborn assessment
   - Pain assessment
   - Postpartum assessment
   - Signs of sepsis (for early detection)
   - Vital signs, pulse oximetry, height and weight
   - Wound/incision assessment
3. Diagnostics
   - Capillary blood glucose measurement
   - Specimen collection (blood, nasal swab, sputum, stool, throat swab, urine)
4. Outcomes identification and plan
   - Antiembolism procedures
   - Chronic pain management
   - Client/environment safety

Box 1-2 Essential Skills for the Generalist RN—cont'd

- Client's activities of daily living (ADLs), mobility, fall risk
- Medication calculation
- Nutrition and elimination procedures
- Patient-controlled analgesia (PCA) pump
- Pressure ulcer prevention
- Subcutaneous (SQ or SC) drug administration site rotation
5. Interventions
    - Bladder irrigation
    - Blood administration
    - Central venous access device monitoring and dressing change
    - Chest tube maintenance
    - Client hygiene, skin care
    - Client positioning, transfers, and range of motion
    - Drain monitoring (i.e., Jackson-Pratt, Hemovac, Penrose, T-tube)
    - Enteral feeding/medication administration
    - Enterostomal care
    - Insulin preparation and injection
    - IV medication (IV push)
    - IV therapy (continuous)/monitoring: maintenance
    - IV therapy (intermittent): piggybacks
    - Medication administration (topical, oral, inhaled, intramuscular [IM], subcutaneous [SQ or SC], vaginal route [PV], by rectum [PR])
    - Nasogastric tube (NGT) insertion and maintenance
    - Oxygen delivery systems
    - Pain management
    - Physical restraints
    - Seizure precautions
    - Sequential compression stockings/thromboembolic disease (TED) hose
    - Suture, staple, and clip removal
    - Total parenteral nutrition (TPN) administration
    - Tracheostomy care and suctioning
    - Urinary catheter insertion
    - Wound care
6. Evaluation
    - Diagnostic (laboratory) monitoring
    - Medication response
    - Telemetry and cardiac dysrhythmia identification
    - TPN maintenance/monitoring
    - Urinary catheter maintenance/monitoring

What steps can you take if you lack mastery in these essential skills?

- Request a review session with your preceptor, who will appreciate your initiative in addressing any gaps in basic nursing skills. Many clinical agencies have a skills laboratory where you can practice basic skills.

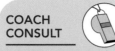

COACH CONSULT

Do not underestimate the impact of doing well in every course and every clinical rotation, even those areas where you cannot imagine working. You will gain critical clinical experience to accelerate your transition to becoming a practicing RN, opportunities to "work smarter, not harder" in preparation for the NCLEX-RN licensing examination, and the diverse clinical base required for future roles in leadership and education.

- Book time with clinical faculty in your school's skills or simulation laboratory.
- Check out audiovisual resources from your school's learning laboratory or library, or request a link from an approved resource.
- Volunteer for community service at a health fair to improve several basic skills in a less acute environment.
- Review related policies and procedures with a peer during clinical rotations. Challenge each other to pursue mastery.
- Volunteer to assist at skills laboratories. When you take responsibility for teaching a skill, your motivation to master it will increase.

Competence

Competence, the next level in Benner's model, develops when you see your actions in terms of consciously devised long-range goals. For the competent nurse, a plan establishes a desired perspective and derives from considerable contemplation of the problem at hand. The deliberate planning that is characteristic of this skill level helps you achieve efficiency and organization. An unconsciously competent nurse may lack the speed and flexibility of a proficient nurse but does have a feeling of mastery.

The "coach quadrant" (Fig. 1–2) explains our notion of *conscious competence*.

- The upper right cell of the quadrant is the ideal. CC stands for consciously competent. You're good, and you know why you're good. You humbly accept the praise that consistently comes your way because of your conscious efforts.
- The upper left cell of the quadrant, UC, stands for unconsciously competent. You may be good, but you do not know why. Your knowledge of pathophysiology, especially, is weak.

WINDOW ON NURSING COMPETENCE

F I G U R E   1 – 2 :   Conscious competence. CC = consciously competent; UC = unconsciously competent; CI = consciously incompetent; UI = unconsciously incompetent.

UC	CC
CI	UI

- The lower left cell of the quadrant, CI, stands for consciously incompetent. Few nurses exhibit the laziness that typically accompanies this approach. Most often, these individuals are in the wrong profession.
- The lower right cell of the quadrant, UI, stands for unconsciously incompetent. Even fewer nurses are apathetic. Most often, these individuals manage their own energy so poorly that they have little to offer in health care.

Another critical point is that yesterday's protocols sometimes become tomorrow's errors, such as shaving every preoperative patient. This nearly universal practice was stopped when it became known that razor nicks created a portal for infection. Broad capabilities, such as knowing how to search for relevant literature, must accompany protocols to have a "consciously competent" approach to EBP.

Valid research also promotes consciously competent nursing practice. Nursing students typically locate and review current research findings to fulfill academic requirements. New graduates can accelerate their status from advanced beginners to consciously competent RNs by reviewing research literature when faced with compelling questions and unsolved problems, such as by working with team members and the clinical educator to update policies.

Another aspect of conscious competence is the ability to articulate a definition of nursing. At a time when many colleagues define nursing as *caring,* we prefer to define nursing more broadly, as *stewardship of holistic human health and healing. Stewardship* encompasses these findings from Swanson's classic 1990 study of nursing care provision, which includes *caring*-laden as well as other value-laden attributes that communicate nursing's domain more fully:

- Caring.
- Attaching (or performing acts of love).

- Managing resources and responsibilities.
- Avoiding bad outcomes.

Consider the following scenario about a patient in a neurosurgical ICU. We direct your attention to the nurse's stewardship of holistic human health and healing on behalf of the patient and his wife.

CLINICAL VOICE: NURSING AS STEWARDSHIP OF HOLISTIC HUMAN HEALTH AND HEALING

Two ambulances transported the Conway family to a community hospital minutes after a drunk-driving accident. Mr. and Mrs. Conway and their two school-aged children had been enjoying an autumn afternoon in a horse-drawn carriage when an intoxicated driver in a large sedan hit them head on. The impact killed the horse and driver and launched the family out of the carriage to the ground. The son landed on his father, which cushioned the son from serious injury. The daughter sustained survivable injuries, including a broken arm. Only Mrs. Conway, who landed in a grassy culvert, escaped injury. The critical nature of her husband's injuries became apparent when he remained unresponsive on the pavement.

Emergency department personnel recognized signs and symptoms of a basilar skull fracture and transported Mr. Conway to a university hospital. Neurosurgeons performed a craniotomy and evacuated a blood clot. Brain swelling remained diffuse, however. They placed a device to monitor Mr. Conway's intracranial pressure (ICP) and transferred him to the neurosurgical ICU. Despite diligent, state-of-the-art efforts, days passed, and he did not regain consciousness.

A nurse who cared for Mr. Conway three nights in a row noticed that his exhausted wife kept her eyes glued to the monitor. The nurse put her hands on Mrs. Conway's shoulders. With quiet determination Mrs. Conway looked up and said, "I know the prognosis is grim, but is there anything I could be doing?" The nurse told her about some recent research that found stroking the cheek lowered ICP, a term Mrs. Conway had come to know only too well. Mrs. Conway turned away from the monitor to her husband and began stroking his cheek. To her amazement, when she looked back at the monitor, his ICP had dropped several millimeters of mercury (mm Hg).

Although her husband soon died from his brain injuries, Mrs. Conway later said that she began to heal when she participated in his care in a meaningful way. She also regained energy to attend to and comfort their children. The Conways experienced a sad outcome, but they could recall some positive aspects of their ordeal arising from nursing stewardship.

The Proficient and Expert Nurse

Benner describes two more stages in the progression from novice: proficient and expert. Although acquisition of these stages is several years away, the terms are worth understanding from the beginning of your career. Desiring these stages and creating a map to acquire them may speed your progression in reaching them.

Proficient nurses consider long-term goals from the beginning, which enables them to perceive situations as wholes rather than as chopped-up parts. Proficient nurses also articulate and follow principles; they recognize when an expected scenario does not materialize. This holistic understanding not only improves proficient nurses' decision making but also commonly makes them excellent preceptors. This additional role accelerates their acquisition of the expert stage.

Expert nurses no longer pause to consider a principle to connect their understanding of a situation to an appropriate action. Expert nurses draw on their depth and breadth of experience to recognize a problem without wasteful consideration of alternative diagnoses and solutions. This recognition of patterns permits expert nurses to grasp unfamiliar territory quickly and to use their repertoire of problem-solving skills to act decisively on behalf of desired outcomes.

Peak Performance Key No. 3: Nursing Process

In addition to articulations of your philosophy and theory for RN practice, professional nursing pride also rests on the familiar nursing process. We revisit its six components because they provide a checkpoint to know your focus at any given moment. Although many nursing professionals pride themselves on being able to "multitask," in truth, frenzied activity is the enemy of excellence. Fewer errors occur when nurses address their patients' needs according to principles of assessment and priority diagnoses.

Many nursing students, even as seniors, do not know that the steps of the nursing process constitute the six practice standards of the ANA (2010). About 10 years ago, ANA leaders added Standard Three, "Outcomes Identification," to reflect an emphasis on achievement of desired outcomes. We value this standard for its consistency with the foundational concept coined by the late business guru Stephen Covey: "begin with the end in mind." The steps of the nursing process occur in a continuous feedback loop, as depicted in Figure 1–3, and the following PEAK Performance Box offers a mnemonic to help you commit these steps to memory.

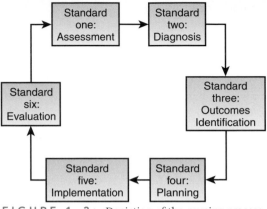

FIGURE 1 – 3 : Depiction of the nursing process.

PEAK PERFORMANCE: ADOPIE

Use the acronym *ADOPIE* (assessment, diagnosis, outcomes identification, planning, implementation/intervention, and evaluation) to promote instant recall of these critical standards of the nursing process. When your approach is systematic, you increase your ability to recognize patterns, both expected and unexpected.

Peak Performance Key No. 4: Best Evidence for Nursing Practice

Best evidence for nursing practice derives from a cutting-edge approach, generically known as evidence-based practice (EBP). This approach received endorsements from the Institute of Medicine, Joint Commission, American Association of Colleges of Nursing, and nursing's QSEN Institute. Although nursing literature promotes an explicit emphasis on evidence-based *nursing* practice, Bernadette Melnyk, a nationally known expert on the topic, reports two interrelated limitations:

1. A sustained research trajectory is required to produce rigorously obtained research findings that are compelling enough to alter nursing practice.
2. On average, 17 years are required to disrupt the status quo to translate a new research finding into clinical practice.

Meta-analyses, or reviews of multiple studies, and randomized controlled clinical trials produce the highest levels of research evidence in support of best practice. Only about 20% of all medical protocols have received this level of rigorous testing and scrutiny. As a result, insufficient research is a common problem in nursing and every other health-care discipline. In 2000, Colleen Goode, another nationally recognized expert on evidence-based nursing practice, proposed consideration of nine sources of nonresearch evidence:

1. Benchmarking data, which identify best practices and include appropriate rates of use for procedures, preventive care data, and disease management protocols.
2. Cost-effectiveness analysis, which compares anticipated benefits with risks and costs.
3. Pathophysiology, which provides the basis for clinical decision making, particularly related to the impact of interventions.
4. Retrospective or concurrent chart review, which assesses standards of documentation and quality of care. Review of individual records provides evidence for many specific patient care decisions, based on known allergies, family history, advance directives, and similar personal data.
5. Quality improvement and risk data, which offer evidence to evaluate and correct specific problems, such as medication errors and skin breakdown.
6. International, national, and local standards, which government and specialty organizations produce to guide practice.
7. Infection control, which applies institutional data to evaluate community-acquired and nosocomial infections, especially when compared with national rates to detect outbreaks.
8. Patient preferences, which contribute to patients acting as full partners in their care. These preferences typically stem from religious or cultural beliefs. Nurses play a key role in advocating for patient preferences, while teaching patients and families how best to care for themselves.
9. Clinical expertise, which depends on providers' capabilities and decision-making skill as developed in formal education and through professional experience.

This second-edition clinical guide and application manual brings you the best evidence from pathophysiology and clinical expertise. Our guidance in assessment, diagnostics, patient care, communication, nursing actions, and ethics will assist you in maintaining a balance between cost-effectiveness and protocols, while simultaneously giving precedence to patient preferences. We encourage you to join your organization's journal club or start one if necessary. You will begin a lifelong immersion in the research process and develop an appreciation for how your organization obtains and applies nonresearch forms of evidence.

Chapter Summary

Chapter 1 introduced you to this book. We provided ways and means to use this guide and developed four foundational PEAK Performance Keys:
- Key No. 1: Philosophy and Theory of RN Practice
- Key No. 2: Clinical Progression From Novice to Expert
- Key No. 3: Nursing Process
- Key No. 4: Best Evidence for Nursing Practice

We included features to increase your grasp of the realities of today's nursing profession and presented bonus material to instill professional pride for your value in providing enduring service across the continuum of health-care delivery.

Chapter 2 gathers road-tested resources from multiple sections of our summer nursing externship and senior nursing practicum. This content will help you to articulate interrelated knowledge from pathophysiology and pharmacology, which will further accelerate your conscious competence. Chapter 2 also presents the emerging technique of dimensional analysis for drug calculations. This approach works regardless of the type of calculation you must perform. We hope you are turning to Chapter 2 right now!

2 Pathophysiology and Pharmacology: Making Connections and Mastering Dosage Calculations

Pathophysiology and Pharmacology: Making Connections and Mastering Dosage Calculations

This chapter gathers road-tested resources from multiple sections of our summer nursing externship and senior nursing practicum. This content not only helps you articulate interrelated knowledge from pathophysiology and pharmacology for common diseases but also helps you make these connections with other diagnoses. Linking pathophysiology with pharmacology in every work setting will accelerate your conscious competence, especially in the realms of patient safety and desired outcomes.

First, we feature some prevalent disease processes that occur across the life span:

- Heart failure.
- Asthma and chronic obstructive pulmonary disease (COPD).
- Gastroesophageal reflux disease (GERD) and peptic ulcer disease (PUD).
- Diabetes mellitus (DM) (types 1 and 2).
- Glaucoma.
- Preeclampsia.

For each disease process, we review the pathophysiology, signs and symptoms (S/S), and major drug classes. Where applicable, we note other drugs used to treat comorbidities. We also provide margin notes, clinical alerts, summaries, and other series features to make these topics understandable and memorable.

Near the end of the chapter, we present dimensional analysis (DA), which we recommend for making dosage calculations because of its universal application regardless of route. DA simplifies medication administration and increases patient safety.

Heart Failure

Heart failure is a progressive, often fatal, disorder of the heart's pumping chambers. It includes several types of cardiac dysfunction resulting in lack of tissue perfusion. The most common cause of heart failure relates to dysfunction of the left ventricle (systolic and diastolic heart failure). Heart failure also may occur in conjunction with pulmonary disease (right heart failure) or in conditions of normal or elevated cardiac output and poor tissue perfusion (high-output failure). Risk factors associated with various types of heart failure include those that are modifiable with lifestyle changes and those that are unavoidable, such as old age:

- Untreated hypertension (HTN).
- Smoking.
- Alcohol abuse.
- Obesity.
- Coronary artery disease (CAD).
- Acute myocardial infarction (AMI).
- Heart valve disease.
- Dysrhythmias.
- Side effects of chemotherapy drugs.
- Cocaine abuse.
- Advancing age.

An important process related to myocardial dysfunction in systolic, diastolic, and right heart failure is the pathophysiological remodeling of the left ventricle. This remodeling occurs with long-standing myocardial dysfunction secondary to AMI, ischemic heart disease (IHD), CAD, HTN, heart valve disease, dysrhythmias, or an aging heart. Figure 2–1 illustrates the cyclical nature of heart failure. Figure 2–2 shows the pathophysiology of heart failure.

Improve your understanding of heart failure through visualization of related pathophysiology. Picture the action of myocytes, brain natriuretic

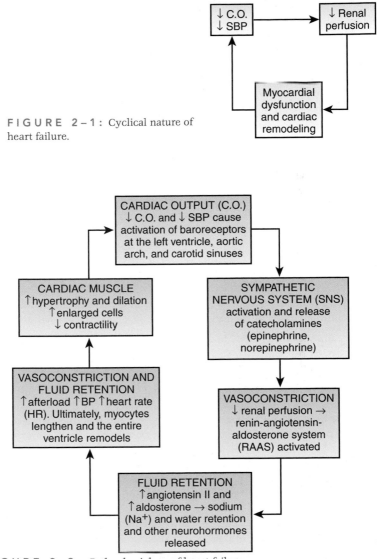

FIGURE 2–1: Cyclical nature of heart failure.

FIGURE 2–2: Pathophysiology of heart failure.

peptides (BNPs), and other compensatory mechanisms described in the following paragraphs.

Myocytes lengthen to receive increased blood volume, caused by sodium and water retention, and to increase the contractile force of the heart as heart rate (HR) decreases. The walls of the heart become thicker in a concentric direction rather than in a spherical or cylindrical direction, which causes the heart to look more like a softball than a football. For a while, this process alone compensates and maintains cardiac output. Over time, increased wall stress results in an increased need for oxygen, and decreased left ventricular ejection fraction (LVEF) results in a decrease in cardiac output.

In addition, various peptides found in the brain, atria, and heart tissues assist the body in its regulation of fluid balance and blood pressure (BP). The heart's ventricles release B-type peptides, or BNPs, in response to an increase in the heart's ventricular pressure and end-diastolic volume. As a result, BNP is a relatively easy way to measure for heart failure:

- Normal value: less than 100 pg/mL.
- Heart failure is just one of the causes: 100 to 400 pg/mL.
- Indicator of heart failure: greater than 400 pg/mL.

Compensatory mechanisms try to maintain cardiac output. HR increases secondary to decreased ventricular filling. BP increases secondary to decreased cardiac output. Other compensatory mechanisms and sequelae include those presented in Figure 2–3. Box 2–1, "Heart Failure Signs and Symptoms," explains the characteristic S/S of heart failure.

Pharmacology and Heart Failure

Patients may be required to take several different classes of medications to manage heart failure. See Table 2–1, "Drug Classes for the Treatment of Heart Failure." They often ask if they can stop any of the drugs. It is important to know a patient's prescribed medications and how they work to confirm the patient's need to continue medications as prescribed. For example, patients may take a diuretic, beta blocker, angiotensin-converting enzyme (ACE) inhibitor, spironolactone (potassium-sparing diuretic), and digoxin. They may also take a baby aspirin or other antiplatelet drug and medications to lower their cholesterol, such as HMG-CoA reductase inhibitor or statin, fibrates, niacin, bile acid sequestrants, ezetimibe, and plant sterols. See Box 2–2, "Safe Drug Classes to Use With Patients Diagnosed With Heart Failure (and Its Comorbidities)." Drug classes to know include:

- ACE inhibitors (actions similar to vasodilators and diuretics): Decrease preload and afterload, increase cardiac output and blood to kidneys.

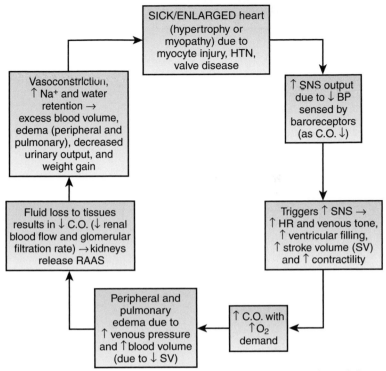

FIGURE 2-3: Compensatory mechanisms and sequelae in heart failure.

Box 2-1 Heart Failure Signs and Symptoms

Know the characteristic S/S for the various types of heart failure.

1. S/S *systolic* left heart failure: ventricles cannot fully contract; caused by AMI, uncontrolled HTN, cardiomyopathy, or valve abnormalities
   - Exercise intolerance
   - Fatigue
   - Shortness of breath, dyspnea, paroxysmal nocturnal dyspnea (PND), orthopnea, tachypnea, cough
   - Tachycardia with increased or decreased BP
   - Cardiomegaly, S_3 gallop, CAD; low ejection fraction (EF <55%)
   - Pulmonary edema (cyanosis, basilar crackles, pleural effusions)
   - Peripheral edema

Continued

Box 2–1 Heart Failure Signs and Symptoms—cont'd

- Hepatomegaly, swollen abdomen
- Distended jugular veins
- Weight gain
- Decreased urinary output, nocturia
2. S/S *diastolic* left heart failure: ventricles cannot fully relax
   - Fatigue
   - Dyspnea on exertion
   - PND
   - Orthopnea
   - Tachypnea
   - Cough
   - Hemoptysis
   - Basilar crackles
   - Pulmonary edema
   - Pleural effusion
   - Normal EF (≥55% of the ventricular blood volume is ejected with each pump or heart beat)
3. S/S *right* heart failure: caused by left-sided heart failure or cor pulmonale; you may note S/S similar to left-sided heart failure as well as the following:
   - Peripheral edema
   - Hepatomegaly, swollen abdomen
   - Abdominal pain, ascites
   - Anorexia, nausea, bloating, constipation
   - Distended jugular veins
   - Weight gain

- Diuretics (non–potassium-sparing): Decrease blood volume, BP, venous pressure, pulmonary edema, peripheral edema, cardiac dilation.
- Beta blockers: With cautious use decrease heart contractility to decrease oxygen demands, improve exercise tolerance, increase LVEF, and slow the process of remodeling.
- Inotropic agents (digoxin): Increase ventricular contraction, provide more complete ventricle emptying, and increase cardiac output, which decreases compensatory mechanisms such as increased HR and increased renin release.
- Diuretics (potassium-sparing such as spironolactone or eplerenone): Block aldosterone receptors, retain potassium, and increase excretion of sodium and water.

Table 2-1 Drug Classes for the Treatment of Heart Failure

CLASS	MECHANISM OF ACTION/ INDICATION	ADVERSE EFFECTS
ACE Inhibitors Benazepril (Lotensin) Captopril (Capoten) Enalapril (Vasotec) Fosinopril (Monopril) Lisinopril (Zestril) Quinapril (Accupril) Ramipril (Altace) Trandolapril (Mavik)	Block production of angiotension II in the renin-angiotensin-aldosterone system Vasodilate arterioles and veins Decrease release of aldosterone	Hypotension, hyperkalemia, cough, angioedema, fetal harm
Diuretics Thiazide (Hydrochlorothiazide) Loop furosemide (Lasix) Potassium-sparing spironolactone (Aldactone)	Decrease blood volume Decrease venous pressure Decrease afterload Decrease pulmonary edema, peripheral edema, cardiac muscle dilation	Dizziness Rash, Stevens-Johnson syndrome Hypokalemia Dizziness Rash, Stevens-Johnson syndrome, toxic epidermal necrolysis Hyperkalemia Muscle weakness, cramps
Beta Blockers Acebutolol (Sectral) Atenolol (Tenormin) Bisoprolol (Zebeta)* Carvedilol (Coreg) Labetalol (Trandate) Metoprolol (Lopressor, Toprol XL)* Propranolol (Inderal) Timolol (Blocadren)*	Decrease contractility Decrease oxygen demand on heart Decrease cardiac output Decrease LVEF Slow progression of remodeling Stop development of dysrhythmias	Fluid retention Fatigue Hypotension Bradycardia Heart block
Inotropic Agents Cardiac glycoside Digoxin	Increase force of myocardial contractility (positive inotrope) Increase cardiac output Decrease elevated sympathetic tone of the heart and blood vessels (previously compensating for sick heart with decreased contractility and cardiac output) Favorably affect electrical activity of heart	Dysrhythmias Hypokalemia Digoxin toxicity: anorexia, N/V, visual disturbances (blurred vision, yellow tinge to vision, halos around dark objects)

Continued

Table 2–1 **Drug Classes for the Treatment of Heart Failure—cont'd**

CLASS	MECHANISM OF ACTION/ INDICATION	ADVERSE EFFECTS
Sympathomimetics Dopamine Dobutamine	Increased force of myocardial contractility (positive inotrope) Promote vasodilation	Tachycardia Hypotension Dysrhythmias
Phosphodiesterase Inhibitors Inamrinone Milrinone	Increased force of myocardial contractility (positive inotrope) Promote vasodilation	Tachyphylaxis Hypotension Dysrhythmias Thrombocytopenia Hypokalemia

*Cardioselective drugs used.

Box 2–2 **Safe Drug Classes to Use With Patients Diagnosed With Heart Failure (and Its Comorbidities)**

ANTIHYPERTENSIVES

ACE inhibitors
Diuretics (loop, thiazide, potassium-sparing)
Angiotensin II receptor blockers (ARBs)
Cardioselective beta blockers
Alpha blockers
Vasodilators (isosorbide dinitrate/hydralazine)

DYSLIPIDEMICS

HMG-CoA reductase inhibitors (statins)
Fibrates
Niacin
Omega-3-acid ethyl esters
Cholesterol absorption inhibitors
Bile acid sequestrants

ANTIDYSRHYTHMICS (USE ONLY BETA BLOCKERS OR AMIODARONE)

Class I: Sodium channel blockers (class IA, quinidine, procainamide, disopyramide; class IB, lidocaine, phenytoin, mexiletine; class IC, flecainide, propafenone)
Class II: Beta blockers
Class III: Potassium channel blockers (bretylium, amiodarone)
Class IV: Calcium channel blockers (diltiazem, verapamil)
Other: Adenosine, digoxin

Box 2–2 Safe Drug Classes to Use With Patients Diagnosed With Heart Failure (and Its Comorbidities)—cont'd

ANTICOAGULANTS (COMORBIDITY, ATRIAL FIBRILLATION, VALVE DISEASE OR REPLACEMENT)

Heparin
Warfarin
Low-molecular-weight heparins (enoxaparin, dalteparin, tinzaparin)

ANTIPLATELET DRUGS

Acetylsalicylic acid (ASA)
Adenosine diphosphate receptor antagonists (ticlopidine, clopidogrel)
Glycoprotein IIb/IIIa receptor antagonists (tirofiban, eptifibatide, abciximab)

Desired Outcomes for Patients With Heart Failure

Increase your overall understanding of heart failure with our PEAK mnemonic to summarize nursing process, use best evidence, and promote the following desired outcomes:

- Assist patients to develop a realistic activity program that balances exercise and activities with energy-conserving actions.
- Prevent edema and its sequelae.
- Prevent or recognize exacerbation of heart failure.
- Understand and promote adherence to all treatment modalities.
- Reduce anxiety about heart failure and its complications.

P—Purpose

- Provide optimal care for the patient with heart failure.

E—Evidence

- American College of Cardiology Foundation/American Heart Association (ACCF/AHA) 2009 focused guideline update for the diagnosis and management of chronic heart failure in the adult.

A—Action

- Foster health-promoting activities, including smoking cessation, weight reduction, and yearly immunizations.
- Educate patients about the need to monitor BP, daily weight, peripheral edema, exercise tolerance, and medication use.
- Explain to patients about formal testing that may be required and understanding the significance of the test results. Testing may include echocardiogram, electrocardiogram (ECG), and laboratory results.

31

- Educate patients to report the following S/S to their primary care provider: dyspnea (on exertion, at night, or lying down); frequent cough; fatigue and weakness; edema of the ankles, feet, or abdomen; nausea; dizziness; weight gain of 3 lb in 2 days or 5 lb in 1 week.

K—Knowledge

- Definition of heart failure.
- Causes of heart failure.
- Classifications of heart failure.
- Clinical manifestations and compensatory mechanisms of heart failure.
- S/S of an exacerbation of heart failure.
- Complications of heart failure.
- Patients at higher risk for developing heart failure.
- Treatment modalities of heart failure.
- Advocacy for end-of-life issues in patients with end-stage heart failure.

Box 2–3 outlines the important NCLEX-RN topics regarding the cardiovascular system.

ALERT

Recognize and report clinical manifestations of digoxin toxicity: nausea and vomiting (N/V), anorexia, yellow tinge to vision or visual halos around objects, dysrhythmias, fatigue, and drowsiness.

CLINICAL VOICE: ACUTE HEART FAILURE AND LIFESAVING ACTIONS

A 93-year-old woman arrived at an outpatient clinic with her son. She had been staying at a residential facility to receive care for multiple medical conditions. Nursing staff sent her for evaluation because of a weight gain of 13 lb in 1 week, which was particularly noticeable considering her normal weight of 103 lb. She also had increased peripheral edema, lack of appetite, and audible oropharyngeal wheezes with cough. Her family nurse practitioner immediately admitted her to the hospital for suspected acute exacerbation of heart failure. She was in acute heart failure and received intravenous (IV) diuretic therapy. The nurse practitioner was able to discharge her 2 days later to the residential facility, on oxygen and increased doses of diuretics. Shortly thereafter, she recovered to her baseline, avoiding premature death.

Asthma

Asthma is a complex, chronic inflammatory disorder of the airways resulting in *reversible* airflow obstruction. The major factors of this airflow obstruction are bronchial hyperresponsiveness to irritant or allergen stimuli,

> **Box 2-3 Important NCLEX-RN Topics on the Cardiovascular System**
>
> - Dysrhythmias
> - HTN
> - CAD, ischemic heart disease, angina, myocardial infarction, acute coronary syndrome
> - Pericarditis, myocarditis, endocarditis
> - Cardiac tamponade
> - Valve disease
> - Cardiomyopathies
> - Vascular disorders (deep vein thrombosis, phlebitis, venous insufficiency, varicose veins, peripheral arterial disease, Raynaud phenomenon, Buerger disease, aortic aneurysm)

bronchoconstriction, airway inflammation with edema, overproduction of mucus, and bronchospasm (Fig. 2–4). Immunoglobulins (specifically IgE) attach to the histamine-containing mast cells or a "trigger" antigen. Mast-cell degradation occurs, releasing inflammatory mediators such as histamine, leukotrienes (LT), prostaglandin (PG), and bradykinin. Cytokines are also released and include tumor necrosis factor (TNF) and interleukin-1 (IL-1). The pathophysiological effects of the release of these mediators produce the clinical manifestations of asthma:

- Histamine causes swelling of the bronchial smooth muscle and stimulates mucus production, vascular dilation, and increased blood vessel wall permeability, called vascular leak syndrome (VLS).
- LT also cause swelling of the bronchial smooth muscle and VLS.
- PG cause pain and VLS.
- Bradykinin causes vasodilation, acts with PG to produce pain, results in a slow-response vascular smooth

ALERT

Ominous signs and symptoms for exacerbation of asthma are pallor, fatigue, frightened affect, diminished or absent breath sounds, difficulty lying down, respiratory muscle fatigue, cyanosis, forced expiratory volume in 1 second (FEV_1, a lung capacity test) less than 30%, and normal to elevated $Paco_2$ (respiratory acidosis).

The following key S/S are likely indicators of the diagnosis of asthma: cough (especially at night), wheeze, and chest tightness or shortness of breath. These S/S often worsen with exercise, infection, exposure to inhaled allergens (animal dander), exposure to irritants (smoke), changes in the weather, strong emotional expression, stress, and menstrual cycle.

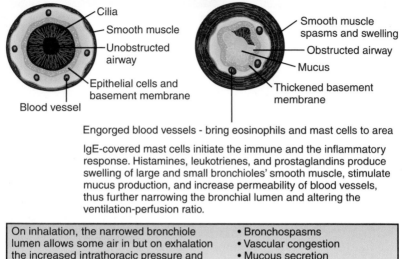

Comparing the anatomy of a bronchiole—normal vs. obstructed due to asthma

Cilia
Smooth muscle
Unobstructed airway
Epithelial cells and basement membrane
Blood vessel

Smooth muscle spasms and swelling
Obstructed airway
Mucus
Thickened basement membrane

Engorged blood vessels - bring eosinophils and mast cells to area

IgE-covered mast cells initiate the immune and the inflammatory response. Histamines, leukotrienes, and prostaglandins produce swelling of large and small bronchioles' smooth muscle, stimulate mucus production, and increase permeability of blood vessels, thus further narrowing the bronchial lumen and altering the ventilation-perfusion ratio.

On inhalation, the narrowed bronchiole lumen allows some air in but on exhalation the increased intrathoracic pressure and excess mucus "trap" air in the small, narrowed bronchioles. In asthma, this is **REVERSIBLE** (see also COPD) but causes the following:	• Bronchospasms • Vascular congestion • Mucous secretion • Impaired mucociliary escalator • Thickening of airway walls • Increased contractile response of bronchial smooth muscle

FIGURE 2–4: Comparing the anatomy of a normal bronchiole with an obstructed bronchiole.

    muscle contraction, induces VLS, and may increase white blood cell chemotaxis.
- This reversible airway obstruction causes cough, wheeze, and chest tightness.

Pharmacology and Asthma

Asthma produces a reversible obstruction of both small and large airways of the lungs. Rapid-acting bronchodilators are the key to reverse the bronchoconstriction that narrows the airways. Anti-inflammatory agents, such as systemic or inhaled corticosteroids, mast cell stabilizers, and leukotriene modifiers, decrease the chronic airway hyperresponsiveness and edema that worsen airway obstruction. See Table 2–2, "Drug Classes for the Treatment of Asthma/COPD."

PEAK PERFORMANCE: USING INHALERS

Take action to teach patients to use their inhalers:

1. Get ready. Take off the cap, and shake the inhaler. Breathe out all of your air. Hold your inhaler and spacer in your mouth.
2. Breathe in slowly. Press down on the Inhaler once. With a spacer, breathe in a few seconds after pressing on the inhaler. Keep breathing in.
3. Hold your breath for 10 seconds or as long as you can. With a short-acting beta-agonist, wait 1 minute for some bronchodilation to occur and then repeat to facilitate greater penetration of the second puff. (There is no need to wait between puffs with other types of inhalers.)
4. If taking two inhalers at once, take the short-acting beta-agonist (i.e., albuterol) first, followed by the inhaled corticosteroid. Always rinse your mouth after taking a steroid inhaler.

Table 2–2 Drug Classes for the Treatment of Asthma and COPD

CLASS	MECHANISM OF ACTION/INDICATION	ADVERSE EFFECTS
Inhaled Short-Acting Beta$_2$ Agonists Albuterol (Ventolin, Proventil) Pirbuterol (Maxair)	Acute bronchospasm in asthma, COPD	Paroxysmal bronchospasm, nervousness, tremors, headache, palpitations, tachycardia, dizziness
Inhaled Long-Acting Beta$_2$ Agonists Formoterol (Foradil, Perforomist) Salmeterol (Serevent) Arformoterol (Brovana)	Maintenance therapy in asthma, COPD	Infection, tremor, dizziness, insomnia, dystonia, paroxysmal bronchospasm
Inhaled Anti-Inflammatory Cromolyn sodium (Intal) Nedocromil (Tilade)	Maintenance therapy in asthma	Unpleasant taste, GI upset
Inhaled Anticholinergics: Short-Acting Ipratropium bromide (Atrovent) Ipratropium (Atrovent HFA)	Asthma, COPD	Cough, nervousness, dizziness, GI upset, anticholinergic effects (dry mouth, urinary retention, constipation, increased HR, blurred vision)

Continued

35

Table 2–2 Drug Classes for the Treatment of Asthma and COPD—cont'd

CLASS	MECHANISM OF ACTION/INDICATION	ADVERSE EFFECTS
Inhaled Anticholinergics: Long-Acting Tiotropium (Spiriva)	Asthma, COPD	Anticholinergic effects (dry mouth, urinary retention, constipation, increased HR, blurred vision), glaucoma, bronchospasm, angioedema
Inhaled IgE Antagonist or Monoclonal Antibody Omalizumab (Xolair)	Moderate-to-severe persistent asthma	Injection site reactions, infection, malignancy
Inhaled Corticosteroids Beclomethasone (Qvar) Budesonide (Pulmicort) Flunisolide (AeroBid) Fluticasone (Flovent) Mometasone (Asmanex) Triamcinolone (Azmacort)	Maintenance therapy in asthma, severe COPD	Hoarseness, dry mouth, oral candidiasis, headache, GI upset
Inhaled Combination Drugs Albuterol/ipratropium (Combivent; DuoNeb) Fluticasone/salmeterol (Advair) Budesonide/formoterol (Symbicort)	Maintenance therapy in asthma, COPD	Respiratory tract infection, laryngeal spasm, headache, dizziness, hoarseness, dysphonia, paradoxical bronchospasm
Methylxanthines Aminophylline Theophylline (Theo-24)	Moderate-to-severe persistent asthma, COPD	GI upset, headache, CNS stimulation, arrhythmias, seizures
Systemic Corticosteroids Methylprednisolone	Severe asthma, COPD	May mask infection; may suppress hypothalamic-pituitary-adrenal axis; glaucoma, hypokalemia, hypocalcemia, hypernatremia, HTN, psychiatric disturbance
Leukotriene Receptor Antagonist Montelukast (Singulair) Zafirlukast (Accolate) Zileuton (Zyflo)	Prophylaxis and chronic treatment of asthma	Headache, fatigue, GI upset

Table 2–2 **Drug Classes for the Treatment of Asthma and COPD—cont'd**

CLASS	MECHANISM OF ACTION/INDICATION	ADVERSE EFFECTS
Vaccines Influenza Pneumococcal	Prophylaxis of infection in asthma, COPD	Local irritation at injection site, low-grade fever, malaise and myalgias, rare hypersensitivity reaction
Antibiotics Doxycycline (Vibramycin) Sulfamethoxazole-trimethoprim (Bactrim) Amoxicillin-clavulanate (Augmentin) or clarithromycin (Biaxin) Azithromycin (Zithromax) Moxifloxacin (Avelox) O_2	COPD exacerbation Classes used to treat *Streptococcus pneumoniae, Haemophilus influenzae, Moraxella catarrhalis, Chlamydia pneumoniae,* and *Mycoplasma pneumoniae* COPD	Anorexia, N/V and diarrhea are common; take with a full glass of water to prevent esophageal ulcers; rashes, photosensitivity; allergic reactions such as erythema multiforme and Stevens-Johnson syndrome Hepatic failure Pseudomembranous colitis
Smoking Cessation Agents Nicotine (Nicoderm CQ, Nicotrol patch, Nicotrol NS, Nicotrol inhaler) Nicotine polacrilex (Commit lozenge, Nicorette)	Asthma, COPD Nicotine replacement therapy	Headache, dizziness, palpitations, HTN; local irritation
Varenicline (Chantix)	Asthma, COPD	Nausea, GI upset, sleep disturbance, headache
Bupropion (Zyban)	Asthma, COPD	Dry mouth, insomnia, anxiety, dizziness

To maintain evidence-based nursing practice, periodically check clinical guidelines, such as the National Heart, Lung and Blood Institute/National Asthma Education and Prevention Program (NHLBI/NAEPP), for new drug classes used in the treatment of asthma. More recent additions include monoclonal antibody or anti-IgE antibody such as omalizumab (Xolair) and a newer inhaled corticosteroid called ciclesonide (Alvesco).

Desired Outcomes for Patients With Asthma

Increase your overall understanding of asthma with our PEAK mnemonic to summarize the nursing process, use best evidence, and promote the following desired outcomes:

- Recognize early S/S of an asthma exacerbation, and understand what to do in the event of an emergency.
- Prevent asthma exacerbations by removing environmental triggers, maintaining medication adherence, and promoting physical activity, while considering comorbid complications.
- Understand and demonstrate skill in administering inhaled asthma medications, monitoring persistent asthma, and addressing worsening S/S.

P — Purpose

- Recommended care of the patient with asthma.

E — Evidence

- Most recent updated guidelines for the diagnosis and management of asthma, NHLBI/NAEPP EPR-3 (National Guideline Clearinghouse, revised 2007, Aug).

A — Action

- Educate patients about the basic facts of asthma (definition, simple pathophysiology, what happens to airways during an asthma attack).

K — Knowledge

- Definition.
- Components of care: Assessment and monitoring, education, control of environmental factors and comorbid conditions, medications.
- Stepwise approach to asthma management.
- Management of asthma exacerbations.

Chronic Obstructive Pulmonary Disease

COPD is a complex syndrome of chronic airway obstruction and inhibition of airflow on expiration. According to the National Center for Health Statistics, COPD (also known as chronic lower respiratory disease) is the fourth leading cause of death after heart disease, cancer, and stroke. COPD causes a progressive, *irreversible* airflow obstruction, often manifested by emphysema, chronic bronchitis, or both (Figs. 2–5 and 2–6).

Normally, the respiratory drive comes from the concentration of carbon dioxide in the blood ($Paco_2$). Patients with COPD live in a state of chronic

Comparing the anatomy of an alveolus—inspiration vs. expiration and air trapped by mucus in emphysema and Chronic Obstructive Pulmonary Disease (COPD)

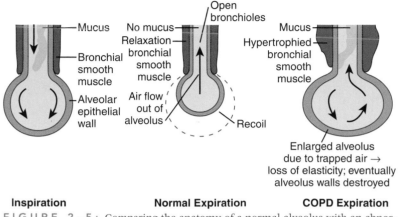

Mucus

Bronchial smooth muscle

Alveolar epithelial wall

Open bronchioles

No mucus

Relaxation

Relaxation bronchial smooth muscle

Air flow out of alveolus

Recoil

Mucus

Hypertrophied bronchial smooth muscle

Enlarged alveolus due to trapped air → loss of elasticity; eventually alveolus walls destroyed

Inspiration   **Normal Expiration**   **COPD Expiration**

FIGURE 2–5: Comparing the anatomy of a normal alveolus with an abnormal alveolus.

Comparing the anatomical changes of a bronchus/bronchiole— normal vs. chronic bronchitis

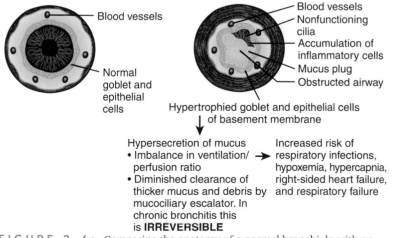

Blood vessels

Normal goblet and epithelial cells

Blood vessels

Nonfunctioning cilia

Accumulation of inflammatory cells

Mucus plug

Obstructed airway

Hypertrophied goblet and epithelial cells of basement membrane

Hypersecretion of mucus
• Imbalance in ventilation/ perfusion ratio
• Diminished clearance of thicker mucus and debris by mucociliary escalator. In chronic bronchitis this is **IRREVERSIBLE**

→ Increased risk of respiratory infections, hypoxemia, hypercapnia, right-sided heart failure, and respiratory failure

FIGURE 2–6: Comparing the anatomy of a normal bronchiole with an abnormal bronchiole.

hypercapnia. Their drive to breathe comes from low oxygen saturation (Pao_2) rather than elevated $Paco_2$. Administration of supplemental oxygen therapy is usually prescribed to increase the Pao_2 to 60 to 65 mm Hg or the saturations from 90% to 92%. Higher flow rates usually do not help, and they can even be dangerous considering the alteration in these patients' drive to breathe.

The most common cause of COPD is tobacco smoke. In smokers, nicotine paralyzes the beating of the protective cilia (mucociliary escalator), so mucus and bacteria remain in the lungs. This entrapment increases the likelihood of infection and further complicates airway clearance. As infection and irritant injury continue, the bronchial walls become inflamed and thickened from edema and inflammatory cells. Over time, persistent injury and inflammation lead to bronchospasm and permanent narrowing of the larger bronchi and eventually the smaller airways. Other causes of COPD include:

- Chronic airway infection by *Streptococcus pneumoniae, Haemophilus influenzae, Moraxella catarrhalis, Chlamydia pneumoniae,* and *Mycoplasma pneumoniae.*
- Air pollution.
- Occupational exposure.
- Alpha$_1$ antitrypsin deficiency, a hereditary disorder.

Emphysema results from permanent dilation and destruction of the alveolar ducts (see Fig. 2–5). An inflammatory process, emphysema commonly results from inhalation of cigarette smoke. Toxins from smoke cause a release of cytokines that increase the action of protease. The action of protease on elastin in the alveolar septa causes the destruction of the septa, reducing elastic recoil and trapping air in the alveoli. The resultant bulla and blebs cause hyperinflation and difficulty exhaling air. This air trapping occurs because mucous plugs form deep in the alveolar tissues and cause a narrowing of the small airways. The action of inspiration pulls the narrowed airway walls apart enough for air to flow past the narrowing. During the relaxation phase, or expiration, the decreased elastic recoil of the small airways, owing to the loss of elastin, causes the walls of the airways to collapse, trapping the air inside the alveoli. Pursed-lip breathing techniques help force more air out of the lungs during expiration.

Chronic bronchitis (see Fig. 2–6) is characterized by hypersecretion of mucus, which occurs as inspired irritants increase not only mucus production but also the number of mucous glands and the number of goblet cells in the airway epithelium. Chronic bronchitis causes bacteria to embed in the airway secretions and diminishes the beating action of the airway cilia.

PEAK PERFORMANCE: MANIFESTATIONS OF COPD

Know the characteristic manifestations for emphysema and chronic bronchitis.
Common manifestations of emphysema include:
- Barrel chest.
- Prolonged expiration.
- Dyspnea.

Common manifestations of chronic bronchitis include:
- A productive cough occurring most days of the week, over 3 months of the year during the past 2 years, without any other explanation.
- Elevated red blood cell (RBC) count/hematocrit level.
- Prolonged expiration.

Desired Outcomes for Patients With Dyspnea and COPD

Increase your overall understanding of dyspnea and COPD with our PEAK mnemonic to summarize the nursing process, use best evidence, and promote the following desired outcomes:

- Patients will develop self-assessment skills of S/S of stable or worsening dyspnea.
- Patients will perform the necessary skills to self-administer inhaled medications accurately.
- Patients will follow their individualized plan of care and notify their health-care provider or seek emergent care for unstable dyspnea.
- Patients will participate in health-promoting activities (smoking cessation, exercise, yearly immunizations, and disease self-management strategies).

The NCLEX-RN examination also focuses on several COPD topics. See Box 2–4, "Important NCLEX-RN Topics Related to COPD." The severity of COPD can also be classified into stages as shown in Box 2–5.

P—Purpose
- Recommended care of the patient with dyspnea and COPD.

E—Evidence
- Nursing care of dyspnea: managing severe breathlessness in patients with end-stage COPD (Leyshon, 2012).

ALERT

Instruct patients with COPD to contact their primary health-care provider if the following S/S develop: fever or chills, worsening dyspnea, increased amounts of sputum or a change in the color or character of their sputum, and worsening fatigue.

Box 2-4 Important NCLEX-RN Topics Related to COPD

- Rib fracture
- Pneumothorax
- Acute respiratory distress syndrome (ARDS)
- Respiratory failure
- Sudden acute respiratory syndrome (SARS)
- Pneumonia
- Pleural effusion
- Empyema
- Pleurisy
- Pulmonary embolism (PE)
- Lung cancer
- Carbon monoxide poisoning
- Histoplasmosis
- Sarcoidosis
- Silicosis
- Tuberculosis
- Diagnostics related to the respiratory system

Box 2-5 Classification of COPD Severity

- Stage 0: At risk—chronic cough and sputum production; normal lung function
- Stage I: Mild COPD—FEV_1/forced vital capacity (FVC) <70%; FEV_1 ≥80% predicted
- Stage II: Moderate COPD—FEV_1/FVC <50%; FEV_1 <80% predicted
- Stage III: Severe COPD—FEV_1/FVC <30%; FEV_1 <50% predicted
- Stage IV: Very severe COPD—FEV_1 <30% predicted

A — Action

- Nurses will assess all patients having dyspnea related to COPD and accept patients' self-report of their dyspnea (measure using a quantitative scale such as the Medical Research Council Dyspnea Scale).
- Respiratory assessment includes current level of dyspnea; usual level of dyspnea; identification of stable versus unstable dyspnea; and related parameters, such as vital signs, pulse oximetry, chest auscultation, chest wall movement and shape, presence of peripheral edema, use of accessory muscles, presence of cough

or sputum, ability to speak a full sentence, and level of consciousness.

K — Knowledge
- Definition and pathophysiology of the group of disorders.
- Respiratory and dyspnea assessment.
- Medications used to treat COPD.
- Prescribed oxygen therapy.
- Secretion clearance strategies.
- Ventilation modalities, both noninvasive and invasive.
- Strategies for energy conservation in patients.
- Relaxation techniques used for patients with dyspnea.
- Strategies for maintaining adequate nutrition.
- Breathing strategies.

CLINICAL VOICE: COPD AND LUNG TRANSPLANT

A patient developed COPD at age 50 years, after smoking cigarettes for 10 years. He was hospitalized every 4 to 6 weeks because he developed frequent respiratory tract infections and severe dyspnea. During this time he was evaluated for a lung transplant and put on the waiting list. After approximately 6 months on the list, he decided to sign a Do Not Resuscitate (DNR) form. He did not want to be placed on a ventilator, which would eventually require his wife and daughters to make the decision to remove him. One week later he was admitted to the hospital for acute respiratory failure. His wife and pulmonologist talked him into rescinding the DNR order. He was placed on a ventilator then and two more times before he received his lung transplant. He has lived with his new lung for 6 years and has felt well and healthy.

Gastroesophageal Reflux Disease

GERD occurs when a backflow or reflux of gastric contents enters the esophagus. Pathophysiological processes of GERD include:

- Decrease in lower esophageal sphincter (LES) tone as a result of certain foods.
- Increase in intra-abdominal pressure because of obesity, pregnancy, or hiatal hernia, which results in the flow of gastric contents from the stomach through the LES into the esophagus.
- Decrease in esophageal emptying as a result of impaired esophageal motility or slowed gastric emptying.
- Defect in mucosal lining of the esophagus.

Intrinsic smooth muscle at the distal esophagus and skeletal muscle of the diaphragm may constitute the entire LES mechanism (Fig. 2–7). Reflux of gastric contents into the esophagus may initiate an inflammatory response, which causes damage to the esophageal lining, resulting in an increased risk for Barrett esophagus and esophageal adenocarcinoma. The S/S found during an assessment of a patient suspected to have GERD include:

- Pyrosis (heartburn).
- Dyspepsia (indigestion or epigastric pain).
- Regurgitation.
- Pain with swallowing or a globus sensation or "lump" in the throat.
- Hypersalivation.
- Atypical presentations, including laryngopharyngeal symptoms, chronic cough, asthma, and dental erosions (Twedell, 2009).

GERD worsens with lying down or bending over and with substances that decrease LES tone or increase gastric acid production:

- Chocolate.
- Citrus.
- Mints.
- Coffee.
- Tomato.
- Spicy foods.

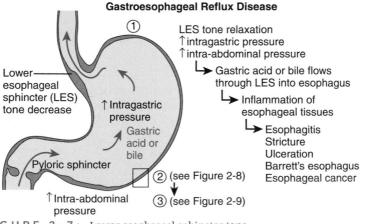

Gastroesophageal Reflux Disease

FIGURE 2–7: Lower esophageal sphincter tone.

- Carbonated beverages.
- Fatty/fried foods.
- Alcohol.
- Smoking.

Foods high in lean protein increase LES tone and protect the esophagus, whereas gastrin, trypsin, and bile salts are corrosive to the cells lining the esophagus. Also, *Helicobacter pylori* and PUD are often associated with GERD.

Interventions used to treat GERD include:

- Wear loose-fitting clothing at the waist.
- Avoid chewing gum or sucking on hard candy.
- Make lifestyle changes (lose weight; eat small, frequent, low-fat meals; separate meals and bedtime or lying flat by 3 hours; elevate the head of the bed on 6-inch blocks).

Table 2–3 lists the most common GERD and PUD medications.

Table 2–3 **Drug Classes for the Treatment of GERD and PUD**		
CLASS	MECHANISM OF ACTION	ADVERSE EFFECTS
Antibiotics/ Antimicrobials Amoxicillin Bismuth Clarithromycin Metronidazole Tetracycline	Eradicate infection by *H. pylori* (PUD)	Amoxicillin: Rash, hypersensitivity reaction Bismuth: Pepto-Bismol contains salicylates (acetylsalicylic acid [ASA]) and may cause toxic levels if patient taking other doses of ASA; hypersensitivity reactions; not for use in children <16 years owing to Reye syndrome Clarithromycin: N/V and diarrhea, abdominal pain, abnormal taste; rare severe—Stevens-Johnson syndrome, hepatic failure Metronidazole: Flu-like symptoms, metallic taste, vaginal candidiasis; severe—aplastic anemia; no ethanol (ETOH) Tetracycline: N/V and diarrhea, dizziness, photosensitivity; not for children <8 years owing to yellow discoloration of teeth and problems with long bone growth

Continued

Table 2–3 Drug Classes for the Treatment of GERD and PUD—cont'd

CLASS	MECHANISM OF ACTION	ADVERSE EFFECTS
Antisecretory: H_2-Receptor Antagonists Cimetidine Ranitidine Famotidine Nizatidine	Suppress secretion of gastric acid by blocking histamine$_2$ receptor site at the proton pump in the stomach lumen parietal cells (GERD and PUD)	Cimetidine: CNS effects (hallucinations, confusion, lethargy, seizures), antiandrogenic effects (gynecomastia, impotence, decreased libido) Ranitidine/nizatidine: Reduction in gastric pH, increased risk of pneumonia Famotidine: Reduce dose in renal failure
Antisecretory: Proton Pump Inhibitors Omeprazole Esomeprazole Lansoprazole Rabeprazole Pantoprazole	Suppress secretion of gastric acid by blocking final common pathway of gastric acid production at proton pump in the stomach lumen parietal cells (irreversibly blocks proton-potassium ATPase enzyme); effectively stops production of basal and stimulated acid release (GERD and PUD)	Omeprazole: Headache, N/V and diarrhea; reduction in gastric pH, increased risk of pneumonia; blocks absorption of some HIV/antifungal drugs; increased risk of gastric cancer with long-term use (in animals) Lansoprazole/pantoprazole: If given via IV infusion, use a filter
Antisecretory: Muscarinic Antagonists Atropine Pirenzepine	Rarely used; suppress secretion of gastric acid by blocking acetylcholine receptor site at proton pump in the stomach lumen parietal cells	Doses needed to treat ulcer cause significant anticholinergic side effects (dry mouth, constipation, urinary retention, visual disturbances)
Mucosal Defense: PG Analog Misoprostol	Replaces endogenous PG, which: Suppress secretion of gastric acid at proton pump Promote secretion of bicarbonate and cytoprotective mucus Maintain submucosal blood flow by promoting vasodilation (GERD and PUD)	Diarrhea, abdominal pain, dysmenorrhea Pregnancy category X because PG stimulate uterine contractions

Table 2–3 Drug Classes for the Treatment of GERD and PUD—cont'd

CLASS	MECHANISM OF ACTION	ADVERSE EFFECTS
Mucosal Defense: Antacids Aluminum (Amphojel) Aluminum/magnesium combination (Gaviscon, Mylanta, Maalox, Magaldrate) Magnesium (Milk of Magnesia) Calcium (Tums, Rolaids) Other	Neutralize gastric acid to decrease destruction of stomach lumen and parietal cells; decrease pepsin activity; stimulate prostaglandin production (GERD and PUD)	Aluminum: Constipation; binds with many drugs (tetracycline, warfarin, digoxin) and with phosphate Aluminum/magnesium: Use if aluminum only causes constipation Magnesium: Diarrhea; use with caution in renal insufficiency Calcium: Constipation; may cause acid rebound; releases CO_2 and results in belching and flatulence Sodium: Affects pH; typically not used as antacid but for acid-base imbalances
Mucosal Defense: Barrier Agent Sucralfate	Produces gel-like coating over the crater of the ulcer, preventing further injury to the area by gastric acid (PUD)	Not systemically absorbed—few side effects; constipation
Combination Treatment for Eradication of *H. pylori* Amoxicillin + clarithromycin + proton pump inhibitor (PPI); or Metronidazole + clarithromycin + PPI; or Bismuth + metronidazole + tetracycline + PPI	Suppress secretion of gastric acid by blocking final common pathway of gastric acid production at proton pump; destroys bacteria by weakening cell wall ("cillins") or inhibiting protein/DNA synthesis (PUD)	See individual medications

Acid suppression is the mainstay of treatment for GERD. Proton pump inhibitors (PPIs) provide the most rapid resolution of S/S and healing of the reflux irritation. As a chronic condition, GERD requires continued therapy to control symptoms and prevent complications. If lifestyle changes and medications do not resolve S/S, surgical intervention may be required to reduce reflux of gastric contents. Antireflux surgical procedures include:

- Laparoscopic Nissen fundoplication.
- Toupet fundoplication.
- Endoscopic valvuloplasty.

Desired Outcomes for Patients With GERD

Increase your overall understanding of GERD with our PEAK mnemonic to summarize the nursing process, use best evidence, and promote the following desired outcomes:

- Understand the definition, pathophysiology, risk factors, and treatment modalities for GERD.
- Prevent complications of GERD, such as esophagitis, esophageal stricture, Barrett esophagus, respiratory irritation, and insomnia.
- Achieve any necessary goals for weight loss, smoking cessation, or alcohol cessation.

P—Purpose

- Care for the patient with GERD and prevent complications of the disorder.

E—Evidence

- Most recent guidelines for the diagnosis and treatment of GERD are from the American College of Gastroenterology (2005).

A—Action

- Educate patients about the facts of GERD: definition, simple pathophysiology, what happens to the esophagus if lifestyle modifications or medications are not implemented.
- Assess patients for baseline S/S; monitor for worsening S/S or complications.
- Educate patients' families about lifestyle modifications to treat GERD.
- Explain the use of various diagnostic tests, including endoscopy, ambulatory pH monitoring, and esophageal manometry.
- Assess the use of over-the-counter (OTC) antacids and acid suppressants and prescription medications with patients and their families.
- Explain that GERD is a chronic condition and that treatment needs to be ongoing and monitored for its effectiveness.

K—Knowledge

- Understand the definition of the disorder and the various pathological disease processes.
- Identify patients at increased risk for developing GERD and S/S of the disorder.
- Know the importance of educating at-risk patients in lifestyle changes, medications, and other treatment modalities.
- Identify when patients should contact their primary health-care provider: continuous abdominal or epigastric pain; crushing pain to chest; pain worsens after exercise; stools have bright red blood or appear black and tarry; patients experience unintentional weight loss.

ALERT

Continuous damage to the esophagus by gastric contents produces an inflammatory response in the esophageal mucosal lining, which can lead to Barrett esophagus and ultimately to esophageal cancer. Refer patients for evaluation of complications of GERD when they present with the following S/S: respiratory bronchospasm, dental erosion, dysphagia, early satiety, chest pain, weight loss, blood loss, N/V, sore throat or hoarseness, and chronic cough.

CLINICAL VOICE: DELAY IN CARE RESULTS IN POOR PATIENT OUTCOME

A 55-year-old patient had complaints of epigastric pain and occasional chest pain. He was an engineer in a very stressful job and had not missed work for a sick day in 23 years. His pain was on and off, and the S/S of GERD had been present "for as long as I can remember." He also had a family cardiac history but no chest pain at the time of his appointment. He was referred to both a gastroenterologist and a cardiologist. He missed his cardiology appointment (because of a meeting at work), but he saw the gastroenterologist, who performed an upper endoscopy the next day and found invasive esophageal cancer in his esophagus and stomach. The patient declined further work-up on his heart and worked for a few more weeks. He died 4 months later in the care of his sister.

Peptic Ulcer Disease

PUD is an ulceration of the gastrointestinal (GI) mucosa from exposure to gastric acid and pepsin. Typically, ulcers occur in the stomach and duodenum. Gastric or stomach ulcers are more common in older men who smoke or drink alcohol or in patients who regularly use nonsteroidal anti-inflammatory drugs (NSAIDs). Rarely, gastric ulcers are associated with gastric cancer. Gastric ulcer pain is often described as gnawing or sharp in the mid-to-left epigastric area.

Abdominal or epigastric pain worsens with ingestion of food. Duodenal ulcers are the most common type of ulcer and are rarely associated with malignancy. Of duodenal ulcers, 95% are *H. pylori*–positive, and the burning, mid-epigastric abdominal pain improves with food intake. Additional S/S are:

- N/V.
- Belching or bloating.
- Anorexia.
- Hematemesis (less common).
- Hematochezia.
- Melena.

The pathophysiology of PUD typically begins with a defect in the stomach mucosal lining. Increased secretion of gastric acid and pepsin and an infection by *H. pylori* (gram-negative rod, flagellated microbe) result in release of the enzyme urease (Figs. 2–8 and 2–9). This release provokes a cascade of events:

- Urease catalyzes the hydrolysis of urea to produce ammonia.
- Ammonia neutralizes gastric acid but is toxic to the lining of the stomach.
- The inflammatory process begins and damages the mucosal lining through autodigestion.

NSAID use may also cause damage to the mucosa directly and indirectly through inhibition of protective prostaglandins, mucus, and bicarbonate. Both of these pathological mechanisms may result in chronic gastritis or ulceration in the stomach mucosal lining. Interventions for a patient with PUD depend on the cause of the ulcer and include:

- Monitoring vital signs (VS).
- Monitoring for S/S of GI bleed.
- Administering bland diet and medications (see Table 2–3, "Drug Classes for the Treatment of GERD and PUD").
- Providing education about the causes, S/S, lifestyle modifications, medications, and complications to the patient and family.

Pharmacology and PUD

Pharmacological treatment of PUD depends on several factors. The presence of *H. pylori,* a hypersecretory disorder (Zollinger-Ellison syndrome), exposure of injured mucosal cells to pepsin, and smoking can

Peptic Ulcer Disease

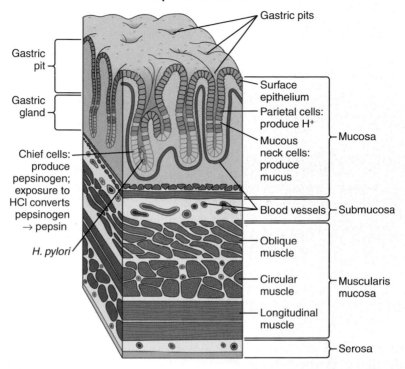

- Ulcers may be due to too many aggressive factors (*H. pylori*, NSAIDs, HCl pepsin, cigarette smoking, alcohol) or too few defensive factors (mucus, bicarbonate, blood flow, PG)

- HCl, from the stomach lumen, erodes the superficial mucosa layer. Over time it may penetrate the muscle layers, the underlying blood vessels, and even the gastrointestinal wall. This can result in a life-threatening GI bleed.

FIGURE 2–8: PUD pathophysiology at the gastric pit.

Peptic Ulcer Disease

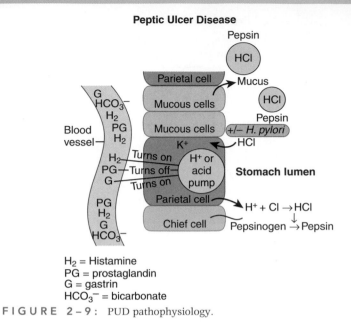

H_2 = Histamine
PG = prostaglandin
G = gastrin
HCO_3^- = bicarbonate

FIGURE 2-9: PUD pathophysiology.

exacerbate PUD. Often, treatment begins with a medication from the H_2 blocker or PPI classes for 8 weeks. Lifestyle changes, listed in the treatment of GERD, are also prescribed. Successful eradication of *H. pylori* infection in the stomach reduces the recurrence rate of PUD from 90% to less than 5%. To treat and eradicate an infection by *H. pylori,* a combination of a PPI and antibiotics is used twice a day for 2 weeks, and then the PPI is continued for an additional 6 weeks. For example:

- PPI lansoprazole 30 mg orally twice a day for 2 weeks; PLUS
- Antibiotic amoxicillin 1,000 mg orally twice a day for 2 weeks; PLUS
- Antibiotic clarithromycin 500 mg orally twice a day for 2 weeks.
  - Note: Clarithromycin resistance has become problematic, and more recent data suggest that a PPI, levofloxacin, and amoxicillin for 10 days are more effective and better tolerated than bismuth quadruple therapy for persistent *H. pylori* infection.

Other GI medication classes include:

- Laxatives (bulk-forming, surfactant, stimulant, osmotic, miscellaneous).
- Antiemetics.
- Drugs for motion sickness.
- Antidiarrheal agents.
- Drugs to treat irritable bowel syndrome.
- Drugs to manage inflammatory bowel disease.
- Prokinetic agents.
- Palifermin.
- Pancreatic enzymes.
- Drugs to dissolve gallstones.
- Anorectal preparations.

Management for active bleeding includes:

- Monitor the patient's VS.
- Assess for S/S of dehydration or hypovolemia.
- Maintain the patient's nothing-by-mouth (NPO) status.
- Monitor serial hemoglobin and hematocrit levels.
- Administer blood products as ordered.
- Place a nasogastric tube when ordered for stomach lavage or decompression.
- Give vasoactive agents as ordered.

For patients undergoing gastric resection, assess patients for dumping syndrome: N/V, abdominal cramping, diarrhea, tachycardia, diaphoresis, dizziness, borborygmi.

Desired Outcomes for Patients With PUD

Increase your overall understanding of PUD with our PEAK mnemonic to summarize the nursing process, use best evidence, and promote the following desired outcomes:

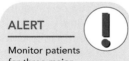

ALERT

Monitor patients for three major PUD complications: hemorrhage, perforation, and obstruction.

- Patients and their families understand and adhere to prescription therapies and lifestyle modifications for PUD.
- Patients resolve their epigastric pain and other S/S.
- Patients resolve their infection (if positive for *H. pylori*).
- Patients are free from complications of PUD.
- Patients' ulcers will heal.

P—Purpose

- Provide guidelines for the diagnosis, treatment, and prevention of PUD and related *H. pylori* infection.

E—Evidence

- Most recent peptic ulcer disease guideline, University of Michigan Health System (2005), and updated *H. pylori* treatment regimens, in *American Journal of Gastroenterology* (2007).

A—Action

- Assess patient history for S/S of uncomplicated or complicated PUD.
- Educate the patient and family about lifestyle modifications to treat PUD.
- Explain the use and cost-effectiveness of various diagnostic tests (fecal *H. pylori* antigen test or urea breath test versus serology or endoscopy).
- Assess the use of OTC antacids, acid suppressants, or prescription medications with the patient and family.
- Review treatment plan for PUD or *H. pylori* or both.

K—Knowledge

- Etiology and pathophysiology of GERD.
- Clinical manifestations.
- Complications (prevention of and treatment) related to PUD and *H. pylori.*
- Diagnostic examinations related to PUD and *H. pylori.*
- Patients at increased risk for developing PUD, *H. pylori* infection, and S/S of the disorder.
- Education of the patient in lifestyle changes, medications, and other treatment modalities (surgical options).
- When patients should contact their primary health-care provider: continuous abdominal or epigastric pain, crushing pain to chest, pain worsens after exercise, stools have bright red blood or appear black and tarry, unintentional weight loss.

Diabetes Mellitus

DM is a group of metabolic disorders consisting of impaired carbohydrate, protein, and lipid metabolism resulting from a lack of insulin, the effects of the lack of insulin, or both. The resulting state of continuous hyperglycemia produces the following S/S:

- Polyuria (frequent urination).
- Polydipsia (excess thirst).

- Polyphagia (excess hunger).
- Fatigue.
- Weight loss.

Diabetes is increasing as the population ages and becomes increasingly obese. More recent DM prevalence statistics from the Centers for Disease Control and Prevention for the United States showed 25.8 million people (8.3% of the population) have diabetes. An estimated 7.0 million of the 25.8 million have yet to be diagnosed (American Diabetes Association, 2011). The most common types of DM include:

- Type 1 DM.
- Type 2 DM.
- Gestational DM (GDM).
- "Prediabetes" state of metabolic syndrome.

Type 1 DM occurs when the pancreas no longer produces insulin. Genetic predisposition and a range of other factors are believed to trigger the autoimmune destruction of pancreatic beta cells. Patients with type 1 DM must take exogenous insulin to survive. If insulin is not given, the patient metabolizes fats for energy, which results in diabetic ketoacidosis (DKA). This type of DM was formerly called insulin-dependent diabetes mellitus or juvenile-onset diabetes mellitus (Fig. 2–10).

In type 2 DM, the pancreas may still produce insulin, but body cells are resistant to its action. Patients with this type of DM are often obese (particularly in the abdomen), have a strong genetic predisposition to the disorder, and are hypertensive and dyslipidemic. Type 2 DM may be treated with oral antidiabetic agents, insulin, or other new injectable antidiabetic agents. If type 2 DM is not controlled and hyperglycemia occurs, it may lead to another complication called *hyperglycemia hyperosmotic nonketotic syndrome*. Patients' blood glucose levels are extremely high, and patients are severely dehydrated. Treatment includes IV insulin and fluids. This type of DM was formerly called non–insulin-dependent diabetes or adult-onset DM (Fig. 2–11).

GDM first occurs in pregnant women during their third trimester. During the postpartum stage, patients may become euglycemic, continue with impaired glucose metabolism, or develop frank DM. GDM occurs in 1% to 14% of all pregnancies; 60% of these women develop type 2 DM within 15 years after gestation.

Prediabetes and metabolic syndrome occur when glucose metabolism is impaired but not to the level of diabetes. Prediabetes is defined through diagnostic laboratory results from abnormal fasting blood sugar

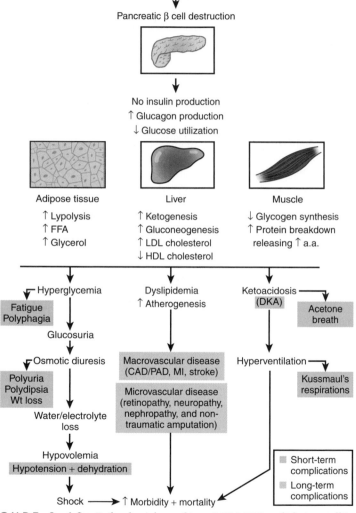

- Genetic predisposition
- Stressor (viral infection, diet, toxins)
  Triggers release of autoantibodies

Pancreatic β cell destruction

No insulin production
↑ Glucagon production
↓ Glucose utilization

Adipose tissue

↑ Lypolysis
↑ FFA
↑ Glycerol

Liver

↑ Ketogenesis
↑ Gluconeogenesis
↑ LDL cholesterol
↓ HDL cholesterol

Muscle

↓ Glycogen synthesis
↑ Protein breakdown
  releasing ↑ a.a.

Hyperglycemia

Fatigue
Polyphagia

Glucosuria

Osmotic diuresis

Polyuria
Polydipsia
Wt loss

Water/electrolyte
loss

Hypovolemia

Hypotension + dehydration

Shock ⟶ ↑ Morbidity + mortality

Dyslipidemia
↑ Atherogenesis

Macrovascular disease
(CAD/PAD, MI, stroke)

Microvascular disease
(retinopathy, neuropathy,
nephropathy, and non-
traumatic amputation)

Ketoacidosis
(DKA)

Acetone
breath

Hyperventilation

Kussmaul's
respirations

■ Short-term
  complications
■ Long-term
  complications

FIGURE 2–10: Pathophysiology of type 1 DM. DM = diabetes mellitus; FFA = free fatty acids; a.a. = amino acids; DKA = diabetic ketoacidosis; CAD = coronary artery disease; PAD = peripheral arterial disease; MI = myocardial infarction.

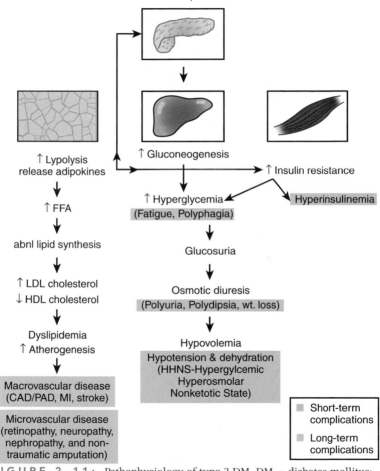

- Genetic predisposition
- Central obesity
- Physical inactivity

Pancreatic β cell apoptosis
and ↓ insulin production

↑ Lypolysis
release adipokines

↑ Gluconeogenesis

↑ Insulin resistance

↑ FFA

↑ Hyperglycemia
(Fatigue, Polyphagia)

Hyperinsulinemia

abnl lipid synthesis

Glucosuria

↑ LDL cholesterol
↓ HDL cholesterol

Osmotic diuresis
(Polyuria, Polydipsia, wt. loss)

Dyslipidemia
↑ Atherogenesis

Hypovolemia
Hypotension & dehydration
(HHNS-Hypergylcemic
Hyperosmolar
Nonketotic State)

Macrovascular disease
(CAD/PAD, MI, stroke)

Microvascular disease
(retinopathy, neuropathy,
nephropathy, and non-
traumatic amputation)

■ Short-term
complications

■ Long-term
complications

FIGURE 2–11: Pathophysiology of type 2 DM. DM = diabetes mellitus; FFA = free fatty acids; a.a. = amino acids; DKA = diabetic ketoacidosis; CAD = coronary artery disease; PAD = peripheral arterial disease; MI = myocardial infarction.

(FBS) levels or abnormal oral glucose tolerance test (OGTT) results. Table 2–4 outlines drug classes for the treatment of DM.

EVIDENCE FOR PRACTICE: IMPAIRED GLUCOSE METABOLISM

FBS 100 to 125 mg/dL
OGTT 2 hours postprandial blood sugar (BS) 140 to 199 mg/dL

Table 2–4 Drug Classes for the Treatment of Diabetes Mellitus

CLASS	MECHANISM OF ACTION/ INDICATION	ADVERSE EFFECTS
Insulin: Short Duration of Action—Rapid Acting Lispro (Humalog) Aspart (NovoLog) Glulisine (Apidra)	Increased glucose uptake, oxidation, and storage (muscle, adipose tissue, liver) Increased amino acid uptake and protein synthesis, decreased amino acid release (muscle) Increased release of free fatty acids and increased triglyceride synthesis (adipose tissue); decreased oxidation of free fatty acids to ketoacids (liver) Type 1, 2 DM, GDM	Hypoglycemia, hypokalemia, allergic reaction, lipodystrophy, edema
Insulin: Short Duration of Action—Slower Acting Regular (Humulin R, Novolin R) Note: An inhaled insulin (Exubera) was voluntarily withdrawn from the market in 2007. Another pharmaceutical company's inhaled insulin Afrezza (insulin human [rDNA origin]) continues in clinical trials during 2013, although the Food and Drug Administration has rejected it twice	As above Type 1, 2 DM, GDM	As above

Table 2–4 Drug Classes for the Treatment of Diabetes Mellitus—cont'd

CLASS	MECHANISM OF ACTION/ INDICATION	ADVERSE EFFECTS
Insulin: Intermediate Acting Neutral protamine Hagedorn (NPH) (Novolin N, Humulin N)	As above Type 1, 2 DM, GDM	As above
Insulin: Long Acting Detemir (Levemir), glargine (Lantus)	As above Type 1, 2 DM, GDM (Lantus)	As above
Oral Antidiabetic Agents Biguanide Metformin (Glucophage)	Type 2 DM Decreased hepatic glucose production Decreased intestinal glucose absorption Increased peripheral glucose utilization (decreased resistance) Contraindicated in renal disease, metabolic acidosis, or concomitant use of IV iodinated contrast dye	Lactic acidosis in patients receiving contrast dye. Do not give 48 hours before or after dye. Does not cause hypoglycemia. Creatinine levels must be <1.5 mg/dL in men, <1.4 mg/dL in women
Thiazolidinediones Rosiglitazone (Avandia) Pioglitazone (Actos)	Type 2 DM Decreased peripheral resistance to insulin in muscles, adipose tissue, and liver Contraindicated in active liver disease, renal impairment, and New York Heart Association class III or IV heart failure	Monitor for cardiovascular events or deterioration of cardiovascular status, edema, weight gain, risk of fracture in women
Sulfonylureas First generation: Tolbutamide (Orinase) Second generation: Glyburide (Micronase, Diabeta), glipizide (Glucotrol) Third generation: Glimepiride (Amaryl)	Type 2 DM Stimulate endogenous insulin production by pancreas Slight decrease in insulin resistance and hepatic glucose production	Hypoglycemia, weight gain, GI upset, skin rashes

Continued

59

Table 2–4 Drug Classes for the Treatment of Diabetes Mellitus—cont'd

CLASS	MECHANISM OF ACTION/ INDICATION	ADVERSE EFFECTS
Alpha-Glucosidase Inhibitors Precise (Acarbose) Miglitol (Glyset)	Type 2 DM Slows breakdown of complex carbohydrates, resulting in a decrease in postprandial BS levels	Flatulence, bloating, diarrhea
Meglitinides Repaglinide (Prandin) Nateglinide (Starlix)	Type 2 DM Stimulates endogenous insulin production by pancreas; stimulates first-phase insulin release typically absent in type 2 DM patients Improves postprandial hyperglycemia Do not use in patients taking NPH insulin; elderly patients; malnourished patients; or patients with hepatic, renal, adrenal, or pituitary impairments	Hypoglycemia
DDP-4 Inhibitor Sitagliptin (Januvia) Saxagliptin (Onglyza) Linagliptin (Tradjenta)	Type 2 DM Enhances incretin system (glucoregulatory hormones released in the gut when eating; act in the brain, stomach, ileum, pancreas, liver, muscles, and adipose tissues); stimulates release of insulin from pancreas, decreases hepatic glucose production Monitor patients with hepatic and renal impairment	Nasopharyngitis, headache
Other Injectables AMYLIN MIMETIC Pramlintide (SymlinPen)	Type 1 or 2 DM Decreases glucagon secretion, increases satiety, decreases gastric emptying, decreases endogenous glucose output from liver Not for use in patients with gastroparesis, on prokinetic drugs, or with frequent hypoglycemia or hypoglycemic unawareness	GI upset, anorexia, allergy, hypoglycemia, headache
INCRETIN MIMETIC Glucagon-like peptide-1 (GLP-1; Bydureon) Exenatide (Byetta) Liraglutide (Victoza)	Type 2 DM Stimulates release of insulin from pancreas, decreases glucagon secretion, increases satiety, decreases gastric emptying	Hypoglycemia, GI upset, dizziness, headache, weight loss

Measures of impaired glucose metabolism imply an impaired fasting glucose (IFG) or impaired glucose tolerance (IGT). Patients are not yet diagnosed with type 2 DM but are on their way to developing the disorder. Metabolic syndrome includes patients with IFG, IGT, abdominal obesity, HTN, and dyslipidemia. The best diagnostic examination to determine the presence of DM is the FBS test. The patient is diagnosed with diabetes when FBS is greater than or equal to 126 mg/dL on two occasions.

Short-term complications of diabetes include hypoglycemia and hyperglycemia. As hypoglycemia progresses, patients may show central nervous system (CNS) involvement and become confused, drowsy, or combative. In the most severe form, patients may have a seizure or lose consciousness. Death may ensue if timely treatment is not rendered or if the body's counter-regulatory hormones are not released.

Long-term complications of DM include:

- HTN.
- Stroke.
- Heart disease.

Microvascular complications include:

- Retinopathy.
- Neuropathy.
- Nephropathy.
- Impotence.
- Gastroparesis.

EVIDENCE FOR PRACTICE: SIGNS AND SYMPTOMS OF HYPOGLYCEMIA

S/S correspond with the unavailability of BS to meet the body's needs and the release of adrenaline and other counter-regulatory hormones and include weakness, tremor, tachycardia, hunger, and diaphoresis.

Review the pathophysiology of type 1 DM, type 2 DM, and prediabetes or metabolic syndrome in Figures 2–10, 2–11, and 2–12. When you understand the pathophysiological mechanisms of these disorders, you can better explain the S/S and treatment plans to patients and their families. When you are articulate about prediabetes, you also may present a more compelling case for adherence to lifestyle modifications. Moreover, you may recognize early S/S of short-term and long-term complications of

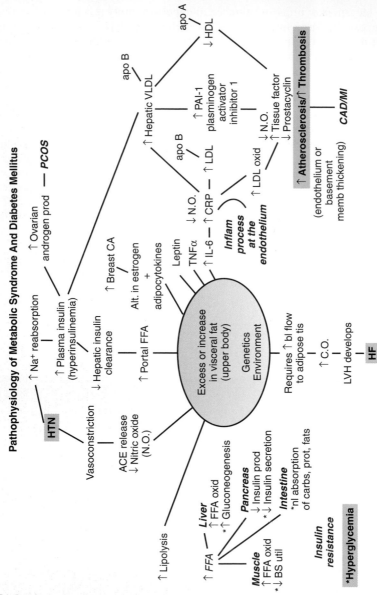

FIGURE 2-12: Pathophysiology of metabolic syndrome and DM.

these disorders and prevent serious sequelae. You will have the power to make a difference in the lives of your patients by promoting health and preventing disease.

In addition, you can help patients understand the importance of tight glucose control. To determine best evidence for practice, the Diabetes Complications and Control Trial and the United Kingdom Prospective Diabetes Study examined and supported tight glucose control in patients with type 1 DM and type 2 DM. Two important current studies to track and explain to your patients are:

- Diabetes Reduction Assessment with Ramipril and Rosiglitazone Medications (DREAM)
- Diabetes Prevention Program (DPP)

Pharmacology and DM

Patients with DM are treated with lifestyle modifications and medications. Lifestyle modifications consist of medical nutrition therapy (MNT), exercise, and weight loss. See Table 2–4, "Drug Classes for the Treatment of Diabetes Mellitus," for medications used to treat the various types of DM.

PEAK PERFORMANCE: SELF-MONITORING OF BLOOD GLUCOSE

Take action to teach patients self-monitoring of blood glucose (SMBG) levels:

1. Gather equipment (lancet, machine, glucose strips, sharps container).
2. Wash hands before and after pricking finger.
3. Calibrate the machine if necessary according to the procedure recommended by the manufacturer.
4. Use the procedure that is recommended by the manufacturer.
5. Record blood glucose result on your SMBG record.

Desired Outcomes for Patients With DM

Increase your overall understanding of DM with our PEAK mnemonic to summarize the nursing process, use best evidence, and promote the following desired outcomes:

- Patient and family will verbalize key components of the pathophysiological process of DM, the therapeutic regimen, and the proposed treatment plan.
- Patient and family will describe self-care measures to prevent progression of the disease and S/S of complications.

- Patient will maintain a balance of nutrition, activity, and insulin availability to promote normal or near-normal BS levels, activity levels, and optimum weight.
- Patient will not experience injury from hypoglycemic events, hyperglycemia, diminished sensation and circulation to the feet, retinopathy, neuropathy, or renal insufficiency.

P—Purpose

- Provide the best evidence-based care for patients with DM.

E—Evidence

- American Diabetes Association 2013 Clinical Practice Recommendations (American Diabetes Association, 2013).

A—Action

- Assess the patient with DM by collecting pertinent subjective and objective data: recent excess thirst, hunger, or urination; fatigue; weight loss; family history of DM; blurred vision; S/S dehydration; changes to skin pigmentation; slowed wound healing.
- Educate the patient regarding risk factors for prediabetes and DM: obesity, inactivity, age, ethnicity, genetic predisposition.
- Educate the patient in the skill of SMBG and how to record results.
- Explain diagnostic results to the patient with DM (FBS, hemoglobin A_{1c}, 2-hour postprandial blood glucose) and related tests such as cholesterol levels, triglyceride levels, and ECG findings.
- Review general recommendations for MNT: moderate weight loss as needed; regular physical exercise; reduced calories; reduced intake of fats; high-fiber and whole-grain foods. Ongoing studies suggest low glycemic index (glycemic load) carbohydrates reduce the risk of type 2 DM and reduce patients' insulin resistance.
- Complete psychosocial assessment and care.
- Educate the patient and family to recognize S/S of hypoglycemia and how to treat hypoglycemia with oral glucose (15 to 20 g) or glucagon.
- Explain the need to treat with antidiabetic medications and any additional prescriptions for BP control, lipid management, and antiplatelet therapy. Monitor for short-term and long-term complications of DM.
- Educate the patient and family about additional requirements of sick-day care.

K—Knowledge

- How a patient is diagnosed with DM.
- Diagnostic tests used to diagnose and monitor DM.

- How to instruct the patient in the proper technique for completing SMBG.
- Pathophysiology of various types of DM.
- Clinical manifestation of various types of DM.
- Medical nutrition therapy.
- Exercise and weight reduction.
- Sick-day care of the patient with DM.
- S/S and treatment of short-term and long-term complications of DM.
- Foot care and prevention of slowed wound healing and amputation.
- Eye care of the patient with DM.

🗨 CLINICAL VOICE: DM IN THE COMMUNITY

Mr. Jones had type 2 DM that required insulin to control his blood glucose levels. His fingerstick blood glucose level was 560 mg/dL, and he complained of blurred vision. Mr. Jones was homeless, and he had not been taking his insulin because it had been too hot during the summer to store insulin and he had no way of keeping it refrigerated or between 37°F and 85°F. Patients such as Mr. Jones need not only more education but also community-based support to facilitate adhering to their treatment plan. A nearby shelter provided Mr. Jones with a cooler.

Ms. Smith had type 1 DM. She often experienced the Somogyi phenomenon, which occurs with too much insulin or too little food at supper or bedtime. Subsequently, the patient experiences hypoglycemia between 2 a.m. and 3 a.m. as a result of a drop in blood glucose levels. When Ms. Smith's BS dropped during the night, her dog would whine and lick her face until she woke up. Ms. Smith believed changes in her skin and breathing caused the dog to react in this way. Then Ms. Smith would complete SMBG and treat her hypoglycemia. She credits her dog with saving her life many times.

Glaucoma

Glaucoma refers to numerous disorders that result in ischemia and damage to the retina and optic nerve. If treatment is not initiated, vision loss and complete blindness may result. The most common forms of glaucoma are primary open-angle glaucoma and acute angle-closure glaucoma. These disorders have no cure, but reducing intraocular pressure (IOP) slows or stops their progression.

Aqueous humor maintains normal IOP and supports metabolism of the lens and posterior cornea. Formation and secretion of aqueous humor begin at the ciliary body of the posterior chamber. Aqueous humor then flows through the pupil to the anterior chamber. Resorption occurs through the trabecular mesh into the canal of Schlemm, with return by way of the venous system. If flow is obstructed at the trabecular meshwork and resorption into the venous system is blocked, the IOP increases in both the anterior and the posterior chambers (Fig. 2–13).

Eye specialists visualize and measure the angle of the anterior chamber by means of gonioscopy to differentiate open-angle from closed-angle glaucoma. Primary angle closure glaucoma:

- Occurs bilaterally.
- Occurs with increased frequency in patients older than 60 years.
- Creates insidious S/S such as tunnel vision, dull eye pain, halo/blurred vision, and decreased color perception.
- Results in IOP greater than 20 mm Hg measured by tonometry.

EVIDENCE FOR PRACTICE

Normal IOP = 12 to 20 mm Hg measured using a tonometer.
Aqueous humor, produced by the eye's ciliary bodies, is blocked from its normal outflow routes and results in an increase in the IOP.
Elevated IOP may cause progressive damage to the optic nerve.

Nurses can grossly evaluate the pressure in a patient's eye:

- Ask the patient to close both eyes. Ask the patient to look downward, also through closed eyes.
- Gently palpate the superior aspect of the orbit of the unaffected eye through the patient's closed eyelid.
- Gently palpate the superior aspect of the orbit of the affected eye through the patient's closed eyelid.
- Make an assessment: with elevated IOP, the orbit will feel very firm on palpation.

Acute angle closure glaucoma is a sight-threatening emergency. Physical narrowing of the angle between the pupil and lateral cornea impairs the outflow of the aqueous humor through the trabecular meshwork and canal of Schlemm and into the venous system, which leads to elevated IOP. Acute angle closure glaucoma:

- Occurs unilaterally.
- Occurs with increased frequency with increased age.
- Causes acute sudden onset of severe eye pain, severe headache, N/V resulting from deep visceral pain, blurred vision and colored halos

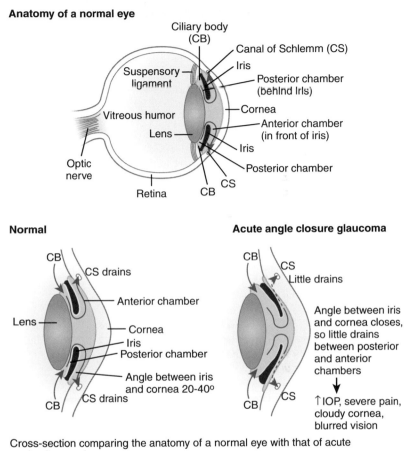

Anatomy of a normal eye

Ciliary body
(CB)

Canal of Schlemm (CS)

Iris

Suspensory
ligament

Posterior chamber
(behind Iris)

Cornea

Vitreous humor

Anterior chamber
(in front of iris)

Lens

Iris

Optic
nerve

Posterior chamber

Retina

CS

CB

Normal

Acute angle closure glaucoma

CB

CS drains

CB

CS
Little drains

Anterior chamber

Lens

Cornea

Iris

Posterior chamber

Angle between iris
and cornea closes,
so little drains
between posterior
and anterior
chambers

Angle between iris
and cornea 20-40°

CB

CS drains

CB

CS

↑IOP, severe pain,
cloudy cornea,
blurred vision

Cross-section comparing the anatomy of a normal eye with that of acute
angle-closure glaucoma

FIGURE 2-13: Glaucoma.

around lights, conjunctival erythema (redness of the eye), haziness
or steamy appearance to the cornea, dilated pupil, nonreactivity to
light, loss of peripheral vision, and nonreactive dilated pupil.
- Is precipitated by prolonged pupil dilation (darkness) and
  emotional distress.
- Results in IOP greater than 20 mm Hg measured by tonometry.

Pharmacology and Glaucoma

Glaucoma is a chronic disorder requiring long-term care. Visual disturbances, whether insidious or acute, may result in visual impairment and disruption of activities of daily living (ADLs). NCLEX-RN topics regarding the eye and medications are presented in Box 2–6. Drug classes used to reduce IOP include:

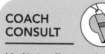

COACH CONSULT

Mydriatics dilate pupils. Both words contain the letter "d."

Miotics constrict pupils. Both words contain the letters "t" and "c."

- Alpha$_2$ agonists.
- Beta blockers.
- Prostaglandin analogs.
- Cholinergic agonists.
- Cholinesterase inhibitors.

See Table 2–5, "Drug Classes for the Treatment of Glaucoma." See Table 2–6, "Drug Classes for the Treatment of Other Eye Disorders."

CLINICAL VOICE: GLAUCOMA IN THE COMMUNITY

After Mrs. Wilson learned about the S/S of acute angle closure glaucoma, she never traveled outside her hometown to visit her grandchildren. She was afraid to have an acute glaucoma attack and not be able to get to her eye doctor. Her family nurse practitioner knew how much she enjoyed visiting her grandchildren and asked for Mrs. Wilson's interpretation of her disease. When the nurse practitioner explained that Mrs. Wilson could receive treatment at most emergency departments or hospitals in most metropolitan areas, Mrs. Wilson heaved a sigh of relief and went home to make travel plans.

- Blindness, causes of
- Cataracts
- Glaucoma, primary open angle or acute angle closure
- Retinal detachment
- Myopia
- Hyperopia
- Presbyopia

Table 2-5 Drug Classes for the Treatment of Glaucoma

CLASS	MECHANISM OF ACTION	ADVERSE EFFECTS
Alpha$_2$ Agonists Brimonidine Apraclonidine (Iopidine) Epinephrine or dipivefrin (Propine)	Decrease aqueous humor production	Headache, dry mouth/nose, altered taste, conjunctivitis, eyelid reactions, pruritus
Beta Blockers Timolol; selective/nonselective	Decrease aqueous humor production	Heart block, bradycardia, bronchospasm
Prostaglandin Analogs Latanoprost or suffix "prost"	Decrease aqueous humor outflow	Hyperpigmentation of iris and lid (brown)
Cholinergic Agonists Pilocarpine	Increase aqueous humor outflow	Miosis (papillary constriction), blurred vision; systemic parasympathetic nervous system responses
Cholinesterase Inhibitors Echothiophate	Increase aqueous humor outflow	Miosis, blurred vision; systemic parasympathetic nervous system responses
Carbonic Anhydrase Inhibitors Brinzolamide	Decrease aqueous humor production	Stinging, bitter taste, conjunctivitis, eyelid reactions

Table 2–6 Drug Classes for the Treatment of Other Eye Disorders

CLASS	INDICATION	MECHANISM OF ACTION	ADVERSE EFFECTS
Cycloplegics	Diagnosis of ocular disorders; facilitate ophthalmic surgery; treatment of anterior uveitis	Muscarinic antagonist; paralyze ciliary muscle	Anticholinergic photophobia, blurred vision, dry mouth; precipitate acute angle closure glaucoma
Mydriatics	Diagnosis of ocular disorders; facilitate ophthalmic surgery	Muscarinic antagonist; dilate pupil	Anticholinergic photophobia, blurred vision, dry mouth; precipitate acute angle closure glaucoma
Artificial Tears	Dry eye syndrome	Lubricate eye; substitute for natural tears	None
Ocular Decongestants	Red, irritated eye	Weak adrenergic agonists that constrict dilated conjunctival blood vessels	Stinging, reactive hyperemia
Glucocorticoids	Treatment of inflammatory disorders of the eye (uveitis, iritis, conjunctivitis)	Halt inflammatory response by inhibiting PG, LT, and thromboxane production	Long-term use: Cataracts, glaucoma, infections, decreased visual acuity, increased IOP
Mast-Cell Stabilizers Cromolyn	Allergic conjunctivitis	Halt inflammatory response by preventing release of inflammatory mediators	Long-term use: Cataracts, glaucoma, infections, decreased visual acuity, increased IOP
H_1 Receptor Blockers Emedastine difumarate	Allergic conjunctivitis	Halt inflammatory response by preventing release of inflammatory mediators	Long-term use: Cataracts, glaucoma, infections, decreased visual acuity, increased IOP

Table 2–6 Drug Classes for the Treatment of Other Eye Disorders—cont'd

CLASS	INDICATION	MECHANISM OF ACTION	ADVERSE EFFECTS
NSAIDs Ketorolac	Allergic conjunctivitis	Halt inflammatory response by preventing release of inflammatory mediators	Long-term use: Cataracts, glaucoma, infections, decreased visual acuity, increased IOP
Angiogenesis Inhibitors Pegaptanib	Wet age-related macular degeneration	Antagonist of vascular endothelial growth factor	Endophthalmitis, blurred vision, cataracts, conjunctival hemorrhage
Dyes Fluorescein	Detect lesions of corneal epithelium	Defects of the cornea outlines by stain	Rare
Antiviral Agents Ganciclovir	Viral eye infections	Inhibits DNA synthesis	Systemic: Granulocytopenia and thrombocytopenia; teratogenic

Desired Outcomes for Patients With Glaucoma

Increase your overall understanding of glaucoma with our PEAK mnemonic to summarize the nursing process, use best evidence, and promote the following desired outcomes:

- Patient will prevent progression of damage to the optic nerve and retina by seeking timely and appropriate health care.
- Patient will perform health-promoting activities to prevent injury related to visual field deficits.
- Patient will understand pain management related to the pathophysiological process of the disorder and surgical correction of the disorder.
- Patient will safely complete all self-care and medication administration (eyedrops).

P—Purpose
- Care for the patient with a chronic visual impairment or a sight-threatening emergency.

E—Evidence

- Clinical Guideline: *Care of the patient with open angle glaucoma,* 2nd ed., American Optometric Association, first developed 2002 and reviewed biannually and considered the current guideline in 2013 (National Guideline Clearinghouse, 1995, revised 2002, Aug; reviewed 2007).

A—Action

- Understand the pathophysiology of glaucoma and its prevalence in the community.
- Obtain baseline data and follow over time: patient history, visual acuity, pupil assessment, S/S of elevated IOP (visual acuity and visual fields, pupil assessment, tonometry, gonioscopy, tomography); administer medications ordered to decrease IOP or amount of aqueous humor produced (mitotic agents, alpha$_2$ agonists, beta blockers, prostaglandin analogs, cholinesterase inhibitors, carbonic anhydrase inhibitors).
- Teach patient and family the need to take medications daily for life, actions and side effects of the medications, and proper administration of eyedrops and to check with their primary healthcare provider before starting any OTC medications, which may adversely interact with some eyedrops.
- Provide preoperative and postoperative care of the patient who undergoes a laser trabeculoplasty, trabeculostomy, iridectomy, or laser iridotomy.
- Teach patients and family health promotion, including going for early detection of glaucoma through annual eye examinations (> 40 years old), wearing a Medic Alert bracelet, and instituting safety precautions to compensate for reduced visual acuity.

K—Knowledge

- Assessment of the patient.
- Treatment and management of open-angle or closed-angle glaucoma.
- Increased risk for drug-drug interactions, including from eyedrops, for geriatric patients with other systemic illnesses.

Preeclampsia

Preeclampsia is a complex disorder of pregnancy. It occurs after the 20th week of gestation and affects many of the woman's body systems. If preeclampsia is not managed, it may harm the fetus and the mother.

Management depends on the gestational age of the fetus and the severity of S/S. The following classes of medications are used to treat preeclampsia: antihypertensives, prophylactic antiseizure drugs, and vitamins. See Table 2–7, "Drug Classes for the Treatment of Preeclampsia." The definitive intervention for severe preeclampsia is delivery of the fetus. Nonpharmacological interventions include:

- Maintaining bedrest.
- Monitoring intake and outputs (I&Os).
- Monitoring BP.
- Monitoring weight daily.
- Monitoring neurological status.

Table 2–7 **Drug Classes for the Treatment of Preeclampsia**			
CLASS	INDICATION	MECHANISM OF ACTION	ADVERSE EFFECTS
Antihypertensives Chronic: Any *except* ACEs or ARBs New diagnosis: Methyldopa	BP >140/ >90 mm Hg Chronic HTN Pregnancy-induced HTN	Depends on class Acts as an indirect antiadrenergic agent in CNS	Depends on class Positive Coombs test or hemolytic anemia (monitor with CBC)
Antiseizure Magnesium sulfate (MgSO$_4$)	Prevents or controls seizures during eclampsia or preeclampsia	Stops propagation of nerve impulses by decreasing acetylcholine (neurotransmitter) at neuromuscular junctions (peripheral); reduces vasospasm of intracerebral vessels	Magnesium toxicity: flushing, sweating, hypotension, depressed DTRs or CNS
MgSO$_4$ Antidote Calcium gluconate	Magnesium toxicity: Flushing, sweating, hypotension, depressed DTRs or CNS	Opens calcium channels blocked by magnesium to allow for impulse transmission in nerves	Hypotension and asystole with rapid administration; depressed DTRs and depressed neuromuscular transmission of skeletal muscle contraction

- Assessing deep tendon reflexes (DTRs) (watch for hyperreflexia and clonus).
- Reviewing laboratory tests (complete blood count [CBC], liver function tests [LFTs], electrolytes for hemolytic anemia, elevated liver enzymes, and low platelet count [HELLP] syndrome).

Desired Outcomes for Patients With Preeclampsia

Increase your overall understanding of preeclampsia with our PEAK mnemonic to summarize the nursing process, use best evidence, and promote the following desired outcomes:

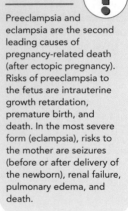

ALERT

Preeclampsia and eclampsia are the second leading causes of pregnancy-related death (after ectopic pregnancy). Risks of preeclampsia to the fetus are intrauterine growth retardation, premature birth, and death. In the most severe form (eclampsia), risks to the mother are seizures (before or after delivery of the newborn), renal failure, pulmonary edema, and death.

- Patient understands the importance of prenatal care and associated diagnostic tests.
- Patient will follow individualized plan of care by maintaining bedrest, maintaining adequate fluid intake, eating a diet low in salt and high in proteins and carbohydrates, and taking prescribed antihypertensive medications.
- Patient and family will develop self-assessment skills to notify the nurse of S/S of magnesium toxicity (flushing, sweating, confusion), following IV load and intramuscular maintenance doses.
- Patient will not progress in S/S to eclampsia (see Alert).
- Patient will deliver a healthy infant without complications to either the infant or the patient.

Preeclampsia is characterized by:
- Elevated BP (>140/ >90 mm Hg).
- Proteinuria (>300 mg in 24 hours).
- Swelling, which may occur and is more serious when it does not resolve after resting, is very obvious in the patient's face and hands and is associated with rapid weight gain of more than 5 lb in a week.
- Oliguria or anuria.
- Hematuria.
- Severe headaches.

- Hematemesis.
- Tachycardia.
- Dizziness.
- N/V.
- Tinnitus.
- Drowsiness.
- Fever.
- Diplopia, blurred vision, sudden blindness.
- Abdominal pain.

Preeclampsia previously was called "toxemia" because it was thought to be caused by a toxin in a pregnant woman's bloodstream. Although bench scientists have refuted this theory, the actual cause of preeclampsia has not been determined. Injury to the vascular endothelium and resulting dysfunction may be to blame not only for HTN but also for alterations in the clotting cascade and involvement of multiple organ systems (Fig. 2–14). Other possible causes include:

- Imbalance between prostacyclin and thromboxane (elements of the clotting cascade).
- Autoimmune disorders.
- Insufficient blood flow to the uterus and placenta.
- Decreased glomerular filtration rate with sodium and water retention.
- Increased CNS irritability.
- Diet.
- Genetics.

The pathophysiological results of preeclampsia or eclampsia depend on the severity of the disorder. Patients may experience any or all of the following pathological processes:

- Hypertensive encephalopathy.
- Intracranial bleeds.
- Seizures (eclampsia).
- Retinal detachment.
- Pulmonary edema.
- Vasoconstriction.
- Liver involvement producing HELLP syndrome.
- Liver involvement producing hepatic infarction.
- Swelling of the glomerulus with decreased glomerular filtration rate.
- Normal-to-abnormal clotting factors.

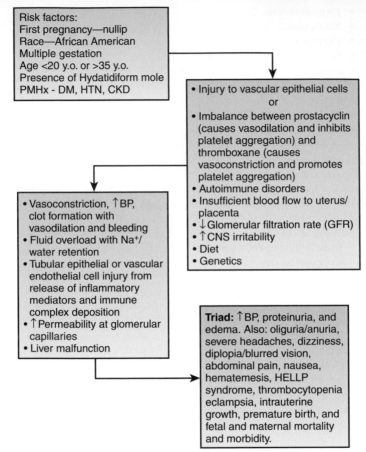

FIGURE 2-14: Possible pathophysiology of preeclampsia.

Preeclampsia occurs in a small percentage of pregnancies. Risk factors include:

- African American ethnicity.
- First pregnancy—nulliparous.
- Multiple gestation.
- Younger than age 20 or older than age 35 years.
- Hydatidiform mole.

- Polyhydramnios.
- Past history of diabetes, high BP, or kidney disease.

Treatment and management of the mother and fetus depend on the severity of the disorder, the gestational age of the fetus, and complications as they develop in the mother and fetus. For mild preeclampsia:

- Put the patient on bedrest, at home or in the hospital.
- Assess BP.
- Perform urine dipstick for proteinuria.
- Assess for S/S common to the disorder.
- Anticipate antihypertensive agents if diastolic blood pressure (DBP) is greater than 100 mm Hg and the fetus is less than or equal to 30 weeks gestational age.

Nonstress testing of the status of the fetus is done two times per week. If the mother's S/S worsen, continuous fetal monitoring will be required until the fetus is delivered. Amniocentesis to assess the lecithin:sphingomyelin (L:S) ratio is not always completed, but if delivery is imminent, a dose of corticosteroids may be given to accelerate the maturity of the fetal lung tissue. In severe cases of preeclampsia, the goal is to prevent seizures in the mother, control maternal BP, and deliver the infant.

Nearly 75% of all eclamptic seizures occur before delivering the baby. Therefore, nurses assess for clonus, DTRs, and seizures in pregnant women with preeclampsia. These assessments provide information about the extent of irritation in the peripheral nervous system or CNS, which may be a precursor to the patient developing eclampsia. Clonus and DTRs may be responses to a decrease in magnesium, allowing an increase in acetylcholine at the neuromuscular junctions. It is not as well determined how magnesium works in the CNS, but it may produce vasodilation in the small intracerebral vessels, reversing cerebral ischemia caused by vasospasms. About 50% of postpartum eclamptic seizures occur in the first 48 hours after delivery. They may occur up to 6 weeks after the baby is delivered.

Indications for delivery in patients with preeclampsia:

- DBP consistently greater than 100 mm Hg over 24 hours.
- Increasing serum creatinine level.
- Persistent or severe headache.
- Epigastric pain.
- Abnormal LFTs.
- Thrombocytopenia.
- HELLP syndrome.
- Eclampsia.

- Pulmonary edema.
- Abnormal fetal HR testing.
- Small for gestational age (SGA) fetus with failure to grow on serial ultrasound examinations.

PEAK PERFORMANCE: TEST YOUR PATIENT FOR DEEP TENDON REFLEXES AND CLONUS

1. Use the rubber percussion hammer to tap the slightly stretched tendon briskly. To refresh your memory about how to find the tendons, refer to your health assessment book.
2. Assess the biceps, triceps, brachioradialis, patellar, and Achilles reflexes. Document your findings using the grading scale from 0 (absent reflex) to 4+ (hyperactive reflex with clonus or rhythmic jerking movements of the limb). "Normal" on the grading scale = 2+.
3. To assess your pregnant patient easily for clonus, support the lower extremity and the foot. Quickly dorsiflex the foot (point the toes to the patient's nose). Watch for rhythmic, involuntary contractions at the ankle and foot. If present, grade the ankle (Achilles) reflex as 4+.

Pharmacology and Preeclampsia

Box 2–7 presents important NCLEX-RN topics related to preeclampsia and risks during pregnancy.

Dimensional Analysis in Medication Calculation

IV Lines, IV Pumps, and Drop Factors

In this section we present the emerging technique of dimensional analysis (DA) for drug calculations. This one approach works regardless of the type of calculation the nurse must perform. DA replaces excuses such as, "I just am no good at math," with self-efficacy and confidence.

Many of today's college students learned DA during high school and cannot imagine mastering multiple, cumbersome ways of old. More compelling, however, are issues of patient safety. With mounting evidence that DA increases accuracy and patient safety, place yourself on the cutting edge of nursing practice through its mastery. Second-year nursing students who were taught DA, rather than traditional math, scored better on a test of medication dosage calculation.

Safe medication administration requires more than rote knowledge of five, six, or even seven "rights." Wilkinson and Van Leuven, experts on the fundamentals of nursing, recommend a systematic 14-step procedure to

Box 2-7 NCLEX-RN Topics on Preeclampsia and Risks During Pregnancy

- Abortion
- HIV/AIDS
- Anemia
- Heart disease
- Chorioamnionitis
- DM
- Disseminated intravascular coagulation
- Ectopic pregnancy
- Endometritis
- Fetal death in utero
- HELLP syndrome
- Hepatitis B
- Hematoma
- Hydatidiform mole
- Hyperemesis gravidarum
- Chronic HTN with superimposed pregnancy-induced HTN
- Pregnancy-induced HTN (preeclampsia, eclampsia)
- Incompetent cervix
- Infection
- Multiple gestation
- Sexually transmitted diseases
- Urinary tract infections

follow for the administration of all medications, regardless of type or route. Their method requires:

- A triple check of critical safety elements.
- Adherence to agency policies.
- Knowledge of medications.
- Knowledge of related patient factors, such as age and weight.

Before you give an IV medication, note particularly any drug-drug interactions and the rate of administration. IV-push medications are typically delivered in fewer than 5 minutes. IV pumps administer medications over minutes to hours, intermittently, or continuously. Pumps administer medications as milliliters (mL) per hour.

Steps in Dimensional Analysis

1. GIVEN: Beginning, what you start with, what is on hand.
2. WANTED: Answer, end with, what you will administer.

3. PATH: Use conversion factors you have learned or can look up to go from GIVEN to WANTED.
4. COMPLETE CONVERSION PATH: Cancel unwanted units and keep WANTED units for answer.
5. COMPUTE or CALCULATE (multiply or divide): Get the WANTED answer.

Example 1

Physician's order: Heparin 1,500 units/hr IV

1. GIVEN = Heparin 25,000 units in 250 mL D_5W

2. WANTED = 1,500 units/hr

3. PATH $= \dfrac{\text{units}}{\text{hr}} \times \dfrac{\text{mL}}{\text{units}} = \dfrac{\text{mL}}{\text{hr}}$

4. CONVERSION PATH $= \dfrac{1,500 \text{ units}}{\text{hr}} \times \dfrac{250 \text{ mL}}{25,000 \text{ units}} = \dfrac{\text{mL}}{\text{hr}}$

5. CALCULATE $= 1,500 \times 250/25,000 = 15$ mL/hr

Example 2

Physician's order: 500 mL 0.45% NS with 20 mEq KCl over 8 hours

1. GIVEN = 500 mL/8 hr

2. WANTED = mL/hr

3. PATH = Have what is wanted

4. CONVERSION PATH $= \dfrac{500 \text{ mL}}{8 \text{ hr}}$

5. CALCULATE = 63 mL/hr

Example 3

Physician's order: Aminophylline 44 mg/hr IV pump

1. GIVEN = Aminophylline 44 mg/hr IV pump

2. WANTED = mL/hr

3. PATH = Given $\times$ Dose on Hand $\dfrac{(\text{Aminophylline 1 g})}{250 \text{ mL NS}}$

4. CONVERSION =
    $\dfrac{44 \text{ mg}}{\text{hr}} \times \dfrac{250 \text{ mL}}{1 \text{ g}} \times \dfrac{1g}{1,000 \text{ mg}}$

5. CALCULATE $= \dfrac{44 \times 25}{100} = 11$ mL/hr

Example 4

Physician's order: 250 mL NS over 30 min; drop factor 10 gtt/Ml

1. GIVEN = 250 mL/30 min

2. WANTED = gtt/min

3. PATH = gtt per mL

4. CONVERSION $= \dfrac{250 \text{ mL}}{30 \text{ min}} \times \dfrac{10 \text{ gtt}}{\text{mL}}$

5. CALCULATE $= \dfrac{250}{3} = 83.3$ gtt/min

PEAK PERFORMANCE: MASTERY OF DIMENSIONAL ANALYSIS

Perform DAs until you master the approach. Then teach a peer or a precep-tor. Would you like to be regarded as a potential staff nurse at a particular hospital or agency? DA makes an outstanding in-service topic during a clini-cal rotation. Track recommendations of accrediting bodies and other safety initiatives for the anticipated emergence of DA as the preferred method of calculating dosages:

- The Joint Commission's National Patient Safety Goals: Goal 3 relates to medication safety (http://www.jointcommission.org/PatientSafety/).
- Quality and Safety Education for Nurses (QSEN) Institute: Safety is one of the identified competencies (www.qsen.org).

Chapter Summary

This chapter presented strategies to connect the pathophysiology, S/S, and pharmacological treatments of prevalent disease processes. Our PEAK Performance approach models how to make these connections memorable for any disease process. We encourage you to implement this outcomes-based method, beginning in clinical rotations, for the dis-ease processes you encounter. This comprehensive and systematic way to accelerate holistic care of your patients will serve you now and in the future.

To conclude our discussion of pathophysiology and pharmacology, we presented the dosage calculation technique of DA because of its universal application regardless of route. DA simplifies medication administration and increases patient safety.

The next chapter focuses on assessment, the cornerstone of the nursing process. Clinical reasoning depends heavily on the knowledge, skills, and attitudes associated with assessment.

3 Physical Assessment Skills and Findings: Firming the Foundation of the Nursing Process

Physical Assessment Skills and Findings: Firming the Foundation of the Nursing Process

As the initial step in the nursing process, assessment of a patient is critical. It is ongoing and may occur every few minutes for a critically ill patient or every few hours for patients who are less acutely ill. Reassessment is a part of evaluation that helps determine the effectiveness of nursing interventions. This chapter accelerates your mastery of assessment with easy-to-reference tables and mnemonics that facilitate a systematic approach. The chapter also includes essential information for a thorough pain assessment. Your patients depend on you not only to address their pain but also to give voice to their individual cultural and developmental factors related to pain.

Assessment comprises two main areas of data collection: subjective and objective. The nurse obtains subjective data by asking questions of the patient or responsible person in an efficient manner. The nurse gathers objective data primarily with a physical examination.

COACH CONSULT
HIPAA AND THE PRIVACY RULE

A foundational principle of HIPAA is a Privacy Rule providing federal protections for personal health information held by covered entities. This rule gives patients an array of rights with respect to that information. At the same time, the Privacy Rule is balanced so that it permits the disclosure of personal health information needed for patient care. We have seen nursing students wishing to share their journey with family and friends post patient

Continued

COACH CONSULT HIPAA AND THE PRIVACY RULE—cont'd

information to their social media sites. It did not occur to them their actions were a reportable breach of this rule. Moreover, they endured serious consequences because they could not claim any of three exceptions: unintentional disclosure on their part, inadvertent disclosure on their part, or inability of the recipient of the improper disclosure to retain the information.

Other types of objective patient data may include monitor readings (e.g., vital signs), laboratory test results, and radiological findings. This chapter presents each type of data collection with accompanying tables.

Subjective Assessment

The nurse obtains subjective history by *talking* with the patient, the patient's family, or, when necessary, the patient's friends. Health Insurance Portability and Accountability Act (HIPAA) guidelines require permission from patients to discuss their health history with family and friends. The responses the nurse receives may be valid, but subjective data can also be incomplete, inaccurate, or false. Subjective history gathering should help *focus* the nurse's physical assessment by identifying specific complaints and associated symptoms. The less experienced nurse often obtains the subjective history and then does a physical examination. As the nurse becomes more efficient, the subjective history questioning and the physical examination may occur simultaneously.

CLINICAL VOICE: THE VALUE OF SUBJECTIVE DATA

As you become more experienced, it might seem as if your increasingly capable physical examination could and should take precedence over subjective data. Resist this temptation, and value both kinds of data. For unexpected conditions, whenever possible, gather subjective data before a physical examination. This order of events provides a second opportunity to confirm or refute related subjective history. For example, a 30-year-old man presented with a painful, discolored thumb. At first, he denied knowledge of the cause and asked only for pain relief. When the nurse pressed for additional data, the patient said, "I think I hit it with a hammer the other day." Murky subjective data raised the nurse's index of suspicion and prompted a thorough physical examination. The nurse spotted a small puncture near the base of the thumb. When confronted with this finding, the patient admitted he had self-injected cocaine. The nurse surmised that he missed the vein. A clot had formed in the principal artery of the thumb. Corrective surgery followed immediately, saving the patient's thumb from amputation.

> **CLINICAL VOICE: THE VALUE OF SUBJECTIVE DATA—cont'd**
>
> The information gathered from these essential assessment activities leads the nurse to form an idea of a patient's health. It is critical to reassess frequently, especially when there is a change in patient status (see "When to Call the Physician" in Chapter 8).

Table 3–1 uses an easy-to-remember alphabetical mnemonic to help the nurse complete an organized and thorough subjective history. Each part of the list does not "work" for every patient complaint or symptom. Adapt the list as needed for an individual patient's condition. For illustration, the third column in the table lists sample responses from a patient presenting with acute abdominal pain. Start your subjective history gathering by asking the patient his or her chief complaint (which is often abbreviated "cc") or "reason for being seen." Document what the patient says as a direct quotation. If the patient mentions other major complaints, screen each complaint separately using the same history-gathering questions. A full patient assessment includes the patient's past medical history, medication and supplementation history, allergies, family history, and psychosocial history. Box 3–1, "Psychosocial Vital Signs: Assessment of Psychosocial Variables," lists key questions nurses should use when assessing a patient's mental health.

Table 3–1 Alphabetical Mnemonic for Subjective History Gathering

CHIEF COMPLAINT		What is wrong?	"I have a pain in my belly."
LETTER	TOPIC	QUESTIONS	SAMPLE RESPONSES
L	Location	Can you point to where the pain is?	Patient points to right lower quadrant.
M	Mechanism	What do you think is causing your pain?	"I don't know; maybe something I ate last night?"
N	New	Is this a new problem for you? Is this something you've ever had before?	"I've never had a problem like this."

Continued

Table 3-1 Alphabetical Mnemonic for Subjective History Gathering—cont'd

LETTER	TOPIC	QUESTIONS	SAMPLE RESPONSES
O	Onset	When did your pain start?	"Last night at 11 p.m."
P	Palliative	What makes your pain better?	"Nothing; I took some acetaminophen, and it didn't help."
	Provocative	What makes your pain worse?	"Bouncing in the car and lying flat seem to make it worse."
Q	Quality	Can you describe the pain?	"It's mostly achy, but it is sharp at times."
R	Radiation	Does your pain seem to go to other parts of your body?	"It hurts a little near my belly button."
S	Severity	On a scale of 1–10, what is your pain right now? What is it at its worst?	"It is about 7 out of 10." "It feels like a 9 sometimes."
	Setting	Does your pain seem to occur when you are in a specific place or doing something specific?	"No; it hurts all the time and everywhere."
T	Timing	Has your pain changed over time?	"It is a little worse at times, but it is always there."
U	Unusual symptoms	Are you having any other unusual symptoms? Do these seem related to your pain?	"I've been sick to my stomach and threw up once. I also feel warm."
V	Valid	Do these symptoms seem real to you? (Try to determine if the complaint may be psychosomatic. Evaluate if dementia or delirium may be affecting subjective responses.)	"Yes, I don't know what's going on."
W	Work	Have your symptoms prevented you from work, school, ADLs?	"I stayed home from work today and don't feel like doing much."

> **Box 3–1 Psychosocial Vital Signs: Assessment of Psychosocial Variables**
>
> Mental Health Nurse Educator Charlotte Spade offers a "cut-to-the-chase" approach for a systematic assessment of essential psychosocial variables:
> - *Perception:* The nurse asks, "What is happening?" The nurse probes, "What are your thoughts about this situation?" The nurse asks, "On a scale from 0 to 10, how would you rate this whole situation, with 0 as positive and 10 as negative?"
> - *Support:* The nurse asks, "Who is someone you can depend on being here to support you in this situation?" The nurse asks, "On a scale from 0 to 10, how would you scale your sense of support, with 0 as everyone you need and 10 as no one?"
> - *Coping:* The nurse asks, "How are you dealing with this situation?" The nurse probes, "What are you doing that helps?" The nurse asks, "On a scale from 0 to 10, how would you scale this situation, with 0 as the easiest and 10 as the most difficult thing in life?"
> - *Anxiety:* The nurse asks, "How do you feel about this situation?" The nurse probes, "How is this situation affecting you?" The nurse asks, "On a scale from 0 to 10, how would you scale your feeling about this situation, with 0 as calm and 10 as terrified?"
>
> Scores are created for each variable and added to give a psychosocial vital sign (PVS), which guides the remaining steps of the nursing process, including effective nurse communication.

Physical Assessment

The physical assessment of the patient should be *relevant* and *focused*. In nursing school, students typically learn an array of assessment skills that are not routine or are used infrequently. Based on the patient's diagnosis and subjective complaints, it is important for the nurse to decide which aspects of the physical examination to assess. Developing *efficient* and *thorough* assessment skills is critical in today's fast-paced health-care delivery systems.

The nurse should do an initial assessment at the beginning of the work shift to develop a baseline with which to compare later assessments (see Box 3–2, "ABC 'Quick Look' Baseline Assessment"): it is *vital* to monitor your patient's *vital signs.* Box 3–2 presents another alphabetical mnemonic to achieve a quick and systematic baseline for each patient. Subtle changes in a patient's condition may go unnoticed if a thorough, focused physical examination is not done early in the shift. The examination and reassessments

---

Box 3–2 ABC "Quick Look" Baseline Assessment

Get systematic! Assess A to E on entering the room:

    A: Airway, alertness (AVPU: Alert? Verbal? Painful stimuli? Unresponsive?)

    B: Breathing (rate, depth, effort)

    C: Circulation (color, IV)

    D: Dressings (check dressings, surgical sites)

    E: Equipment/environment (check pumps, tubes, chest tubes; assess environment for warmth, lights on, shades drawn, clutter, safety)

Assess F to I at the bedside:

    F: Facts/feeling: How is the patient feeling? How was the patient's day/night? Does the patient have pain? What are the patient's needs this shift?

    G: Get vital signs: Look, listen, and feel

    H: Head to toe: Any emergency findings at any point in your assessment? Go to I.

    I: Intervene

---

should be *prioritized and systematic. Inspection* is a critical part of the physical examination and should be done in conjunction with *palpation* and *auscultation.* Percussion is used much less often.

Table 3–2, "Alphabetical Mnemonic for Systematic Physical and Room Assessment," presents a guide to conducting a focused physical examination with emphasis on the following systems: respiratory, cardiovascular, gastrointestinal/genitourinary (GI/GU), neurological, and musculoskeletal/skin. In addition to assessing the patient, the nurse should "assess" the room as an extension of the patient's physical systems.

Table 3–3 lists typical assessment techniques and normal and abnormal documentation findings for the major body systems.

Table 3–4 lists the 12 cranial nerves, a basic evaluation of each nerve, and a brief listing of normal and abnormal findings.

The skin is the largest organ of the body, and the nurse may need to document lesions that develop on a patient's skin or monitor existing lesions. Lesions are any pathological change in normal tissue. Common examples include lacerations, incisions, rashes, moles, and ulcers. The nurse assessing a lesion should use the mnemonic "cuts-n-rashes" to evaluate the lesion's characteristics. Table 3–5, "Cuts-n-Rashes: A Skin Assessment Mnemonic and Lesion Example," lists these characteristics with a brief explanation and sample documentation (based on Fig. 3–4). Patients

(Text continues on page 102)

Table 3–2 Alphabetical Mnemonic for Systematic Physical and Room Assessment

SYSTEM	PHYSICAL EXAMINATION SKILLS	ADDITIONAL ROOM ASSESSMENT
Airway	*Inspect:* Patent and unobstructed airway *Listen:* Is the patient talking? Is there stridor? Do you feel air movement from the patient's mouth or nose?	Verify suction ready for removing secretions or emesis
Breathing	*Inspect* and *palpate:* Work of breathing—evaluate rate and rhythm; skin temperature and moisture—rise and fall of chest; abnormalities *Auscultate:* Listen with diaphragm over posterior and anterior; upper, mid, and lower lobes; alternating side-to-side, through a complete inspiration and expiration cycle; document rate, rhythm, normal sounds, abnormal sounds (Fig. 3–1) 	Oxygen equipment: correct amount of oxygen and delivery device (cannula, mask, bag-valve mask)

FIGURE 3–1: *A*, Anterior respiratory auscultation sites.

Table 3–2 Alphabetical Mnemonic for Systematic Physical and Room Assessment—cont'd

SYSTEM	PHYSICAL EXAMINATION SKILLS	ADDITIONAL ROOM ASSESSMENT
	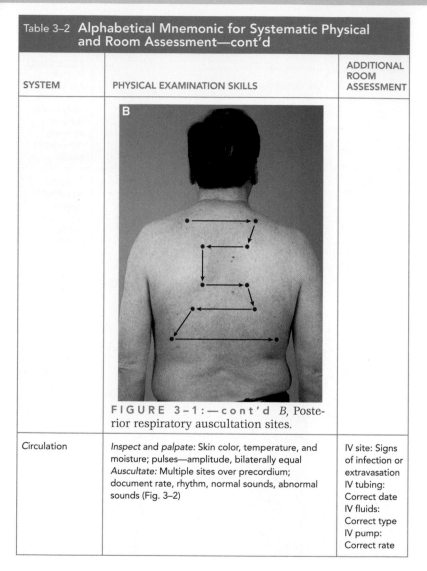 FIGURE 3–1:—cont'd *B*, Posterior respiratory auscultation sites.	
Circulation	*Inspect* and *palpate:* Skin color, temperature, and moisture; pulses—amplitude, bilaterally equal *Auscultate:* Multiple sites over precordium; document rate, rhythm, normal sounds, abnormal sounds (Fig. 3–2)	IV site: Signs of infection or extravasation IV tubing: Correct date IV fluids: Correct type IV pump: Correct rate

Table 3-2 Alphabetical Mnemonic for Systematic Physical and Room Assessment—cont'd

SYSTEM	PHYSICAL EXAMINATION SKILLS	ADDITIONAL ROOM ASSESSMENT
	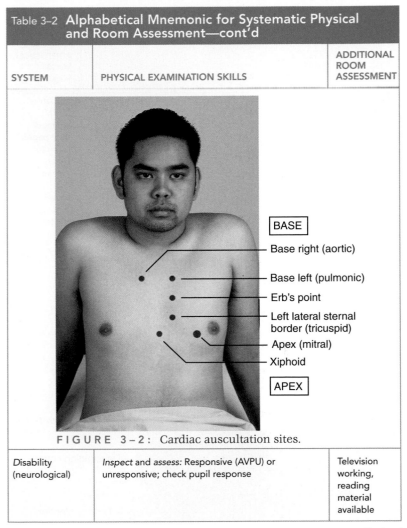 BASE — Base right (aortic) — Base left (pulmonic) — Erb's point — Left lateral sternal border (tricuspid) — Apex (mitral) — Xiphoid APEX FIGURE 3-2: Cardiac auscultation sites.	
Disability (neurological)	*Inspect* and *assess:* Responsive (AVPU) or unresponsive; check pupil response	Television working, reading material available

Continued

		ADDITIONAL ROOM ASSESSMENT
Table 3–2 Alphabetical Mnemonic for Systematic Physical and Room Assessment—cont'd		
SYSTEM	PHYSICAL EXAMINATION SKILLS	
Digestion (GI/GU)	*Auscultate:* Bowel sounds throughout abdomen *Palpate:* Check for tenderness (rebound), distention, or masses (Fig. 3–3)	Bedpan, urinal, commode, toilet paper available Urinary drainage system functions Urine amount and color

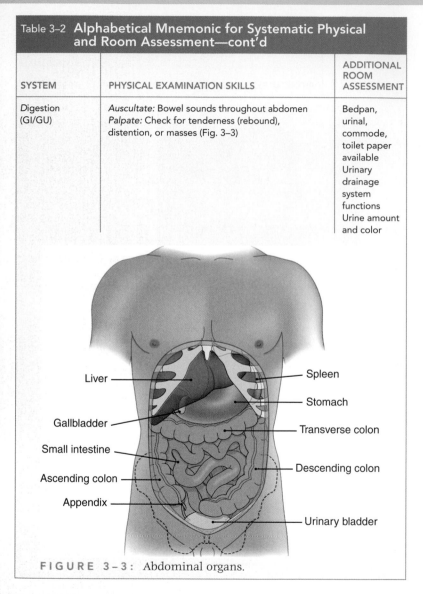

FIGURE 3-3: Abdominal organs.

Table 3–2 Alphabetical Mnemonic for Systematic Physical and Room Assessment—cont'd

SYSTEM	PHYSICAL EXAMINATION SKILLS	ADDITIONAL ROOM ASSESSMENT
External (musculoskeletal and skin)	*Musculoskeletal—inspect* and *palpate*: Joint range of motion (ROM), extremity circulation, movement, and sensation (CMS) *Skin—inspect* and *palpate*: Skin—temperature, texture, turgor, and moisture; lesions, wounds, incisions—color, elevation, pattern or shape, size (cm), location and distribution, exudate (color, consistency, amount)	Trapeze Antiembolism devices Pressure point devices: Special mattresses, heel/elbow cups Lotion

Table 3–3 Assessment Techniques and Documentation Findings

EXAMINATION	NORMAL FINDINGS	ABNORMAL FINDINGS
Head, Eyes, Ears, Nose, Throat (HEENT)		
Inspect and Palpate Bony structures and soft tissues of the head	**HEAD** Normocephalic Atraumatic	Micro/macrocephalic Lesions (wounds, rash) Infestations (lice, fungus)
Inspect and Test Pupil size, shape, reactivity to light Conjunctiva Extraocular muscle function (EOM) Visual acuity	**EYES** Pupils equal, round, reactive to light (PERRL) Clear EOM intact 20/20 in both eyes	Mydriasis, miosis, anisocoria Ptosis Injected, chemosis Strabismus, nystagmus
Inspect and Palpate Auricle/tragus: Size, shape, tenderness Whisper test	**EARS** External ears atraumatic and nontender; canals clear, without exudates; hearing grossly intact; patient responds appropriately to questions	Tragal tenderness Bloody/cerebrospinal fluid (CSF) drainage Diminished hearing

Continued

95

Table 3–3	Assessment Techniques and Documentation Findings—cont'd	
EXAMINATION	NORMAL FINDINGS	ABNORMAL FINDINGS
Head, Eyes, Ears, Nose, Throat (HEENT)—cont'd		
Inspect and Palpate Bony structures and soft tissues of the nose	**NOSE** Midline atraumatic, without tenderness or exudate	Deviated septum Anosmia Polyps Discolored or excessive exudate
Inspect Lips, oral and buccal mucosa, gums, teeth, tongue, floor of mouth, pharynx *Test* Tongue strength/ protrusion	**THROAT** Pink and moist without lesions Midline	Erythema, edema, exudates, caries, lesions Deviation to one side or decreased strength
Neck		
Inspect and Palpate Lymph nodes Thyroid Trachea Jugular veins *Palpate and Auscultate* Carotid arteries	Nontender, mobile, not enlarged Nontender, not enlarged Midline Nondistended Regular rhythm	Tender, fixed, lymphadenopathy Goiter, nodules Deviated Distended Bruits, bigeminal pulse, thrill
Thorax and Lungs		
Inspect and Palpate Chest wall/skin Respiratory effort *Auscultate* Posterior and anterior lung lobes	Anterior-posterior: Transverse diameter (AP:T) = 1:2, skin warm, moist without cyanosis or lesions Eupnea Lung sounds clear to auscultation, equal, with adequate aeration, bilaterally	Barrel chest, deformity, or asymmetry; subcutaneous emphysema; cyanosis; nail clubbing Retractions, accessory muscle use, increased work of breathing, dyspnea, bradypnea, tachypnea Rales (crackles), rhonchi, wheezes, stridor, diminished breath sounds/aeration

Table 3–3 Assessment Techniques and Documentation Findings—cont'd

EXAMINATION	NORMAL FINDINGS	ABNORMAL FINDINGS
Cardiovascular		
Inspect and Palpate Peripheral pulses Precordium, apical impulse *Auscultate* Precordium sites	Equal, 2+ amplitude, bilaterally Regular rate and rhythm, S_1 and S_2, without murmurs, rubs, gallops, or splits	Diminished, pulsus alternans, bigeminal pulse, paradoxical pulse Lifts, heaves, thrills Irregular rhythm, S_3, S_4, murmurs, pericardial friction rub, splits
GI/GU		
Inspect Abdominal wall/skin *Auscultate* Bowel sounds *Palpate* Abdominal organs *Percuss* Costovertebral angle	Flat, nondistended, without lesions All four quadrants normoactive Nontender, without organomegaly Nontender	Scaphoid, distended, obese Hyperactive, hypoactive, borborygmi Positive McBurney point tenderness, inspiratory arrest, rigid, hepatomegaly, splenomegaly Positive costovertebral angle tenderness
Neurological		
Inspect and Assess Mental status (Mini-Mental State Exam, Glasgow Coma Scale) Cranial nerves (see Table 3–4) Sensation (sharp and dull) Coordination Deep tendon reflexes (DTR) 5+ = Sustained clonus 4+ = Very brisk, hyperreflexive, with clonus 3+ = Brisker or more reflexive than normal 2+ = Normal amount of reflex 1+ = Low normal, diminished reflex	Mental status examination shows appropriate speech, behavior, and appearance; alert and oriented (A&O) × 3 (to person, place, and time) with intact recent and remote memory Cranial nerves II–XII grossly intact Sharp and dull correctly identified on all extremities Range of motion (ROM) without deficit, negative for Romberg sign, negative for pronator drift Smooth, even gait	Slurred speech, disheveled clothing, poor hygiene; A&O × 1 to name only; memory test responses inaccurate See Table 3–4 Diminished sharp or dull perception in distal feet bilaterally Spastic gait with uncoordinated ROM; positive for Romberg's sign Hyperreflexive (4+) right patellar DTR

Continued

Table 3–3 Assessment Techniques and Documentation Findings—cont'd

EXAMINATION	NORMAL FINDINGS	ABNORMAL FINDINGS
Neurological—cont'd		
0.5+ = Reflex elicited only with reinforcement 0 = No response	DTR 2+ (normal amount of reflex) bilaterally	
Musculoskeletal		
Inspect, Palpate, and Test Upper and lower extremities/joints, back (strength and range of motion [ROM])	Full, active ROM; strength +5/5	Edema, decreased ROM/strength, crepitus
Integumentary		
Inspect and Palpate Skin Color, temperature, turgor, moisture Check lesions/wounds for color, elevation, pattern or shape, size (cm), location and distribution, exudate (color, consistency, amount) (see Table 3–5)	Coloration normal for race, warm, dry; elastic turgor	Pale, cyanotic, tenting turgor

Table 3–4 Cranial Nerves

CRANIAL NERVE NUMBER, NAME[1] (FUNCTION[2])	BASIC TESTING	NORMAL FINDINGS[2]	ABNORMAL FINDINGS
I, Olfactory (S)	Occlude each naris; test smell with two familiar, distinct, nonirritating scents (coffee, soap) [rarely tested]	Intact bilaterally (B)	Anosmia
II, Optic (S)	Snellen eye chart or pocket vision screening	20/20 OU	Diminished vision

Table 3–4 Cranial Nerves—cont'd

CRANIAL NERVE NUMBER, NAME[1] (FUNCTION[2])	BASIC TESTING	NORMAL FINDINGS[2]	ABNORMAL FINDINGS
III, Oculomotor (M)	Motor (M): Extra ocular movement Sensory (S): Shine light in pupil	M: Equal OU movement to medial, upper inner, outer, and lower outer areas S: Equal OU light reflex	M: Ptosis, strabismus, nystagmus S: Nonresponsive light reflex
IV, Trochlear (M)	Extraocular motor (EOM) movement	Down and inward OU movement	Incorrect movement
V, Trigeminal (B)	M: Palpate for masseter and temporalis muscle contraction with hands S: Test and compare light touch to forehead, cheek, and chin bilaterally	M: Strong contraction with teeth clenching S: Positive sensation in all three branches (B)	M: Diminished or absent contraction S: Loss of sensation in one or more branches
VI, Abducens (M)	EOM movement	Lateral OU movement	Incorrect movement
VII, Facial (B)	M: Ask patient to smile, frown, close eyes tightly, purse lips and puff cheeks, show teeth S: Test taste in anterior two-thirds of tongue [rarely tested]	M: Facial movements intact (B) S: Sweet, sour, salty taste intact (B)	M: Diminished or absent facial movements S: Diminished or absent taste
VIII, Acoustic (S)	Evaluate ability to hear whisper or snapping fingers in each ear	Hearing grossly intact (B)	Diminished hearing

Continued

99

Table 3–4 Cranial Nerves—cont'd

CRANIAL NERVE NUMBER, NAME[1] (FUNCTION[2])	BASIC TESTING	NORMAL FINDINGS[2]	ABNORMAL FINDINGS
IX, Glossopharyngeal (B) X, Vagus (B)	M: Evaluate speech, swallowing, and uvula rising when patient says "ah" S: Test taste in posterior third of tongue [rarely tested]	M: Clear speech with uvula rising midline; positive gag reflex S: Sweet, sour, salty taste intact (B)	M: Voice changes, uvula rises to one side, dysphagia or absent gag reflex S: Diminished or absent taste
XI, Spinal accessory (M)	Have patient shrug shoulders and move head side to side against resistance	Symmetrical, strong movements	Diminished strength or unequal movement
XII, Hypoglossal (M)	Evaluate speech; protrude tongue and move side to side	Clear, articulate speech; tongue protrudes midline	Dysarthria; tongue protrudes to one side

[1]Sample mnemonic for remembering cranial nerves: On Old Olympus Towering Tops A Finn And German Viewed Some Hops

[2]Sample mnemonic for remembering whether each cranial nerve has sensory (S), motor (M), or both (B) functions: Some Say Marry Money But My Brother Says Bad Business Marry Money

Table 3–5 Cuts-n-Rashes: A Skin Assessment Mnemonic and Lesion Example

MNEMONIC AND LESION CHARACTERISTIC	SAMPLE DOCUMENTATION
Color: Describe lesions' shades of color and note changing color over time	Centralized blackened area with dark erythematous border and mild erythema out to 7 cm
Unusual symptoms: Ask patient if experiencing any systemic symptoms; these may be due to the lesions (e.g., fever, malaise)	Patient complains of recent generalized malaise and achiness
Texture: Palpate the lesions' texture; how do the lesions feel?	Rough texture in central area

Table 3–5 **Cuts-n-Rashes: A Skin Assessment Mnemonic and Lesion Example—cont'd**

MNEMONIC AND LESION CHARACTERISTIC	SAMPLE DOCUMENTATION
Shape: Describe the lesions' shape	Generally circular
Noxious: Are the lesions itchy? Painful?	Patient complains of mild itchiness and moderate tenderness
Reason: Does the patient know what caused the lesions?	Patient states "bitten by a spider"
Area: Describe location and distribution of the lesions	Right posterior calf
Size: Measured in cm or mm	Central area blackened ~0.5 cm in diameter with erythematous border 1 cm; mild erythema extends 7 cm out from lesion
Height: Are the lesions elevated above the skin? How deep are they?	Central area elevated ~0.25 cm
Exudate: Describe any drainage—type, color, consistency, and quantity	Small amount of purulent exudate from central lesion
Smell: Do the lesions or drainage have an odor?	No noticeable odor

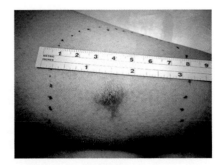

FIGURE 3–4: Example of a lower leg lesion.

with dark skin (African Americans) may present with lesions with characteristics different from lesions of light-skinned patients. Erythema, a typical sign of infection, may be difficult to assess in dark skin, and the nurse may need to evaluate other typical characteristics of infection (increased skin temperature, localized edema and tenderness, purulent exudate). Dark-colored skin often appears ashen-gray or dusky and loses its shiny texture when circulation to an area is decreased. Nurses working with populations having a range of skin coloration need to learn wound and lesion assessment skills through experience and the mentoring of more experienced nurses.

Pain Assessment

Pain is referred to as the "fifth vital sign," and its assessment is an expected and routine part of patient assessment. The standard of the Joint Commission (JC) regarding pain assessment states: "A comprehensive pain assessment is conducted as appropriate to the individual's condition and the scope of care, treatment and services provided" (JC, 2008, Paragraph 2). The JC reaffirmed this standard in 2012. The nurse is responsible for determining an appropriate frequency of assessing pain based on agency policy and each patient's unique condition. When pain medication is administered, the nurse is responsible for reassessing the pain level as well as monitoring for side effects of medication, such as slowed respirations.

Pain is a subjective finding, and the nurse should be aware that the patient is the authority on his or her pain and is the only one who can define the pain experience. The nurse must rely on the patient's *words* and *behaviors* to understand that individual's pain experience. The response to pain is influenced by past personal experiences and by social and cultural factors. For example, frequent painful procedures in infants may alter the child's pain response for the rest of his or her life. Long-term consequences for infants who had repetitive and poorly controlled pain include

> **ALERT**
>
> The ABCs of PAIN MANAGEMENT
>
> A—Ask about pain regularly; assess pain systematically.
> B—Believe the patient and family in their reports of pain and what relieves it.
> C—Choose pain control options appropriate for the patient, family, and setting.
> D—Deliver interventions in a timely, logical, and coordinated fashion.
> E—Empower patients and their families; enable patients to control their course to the greatest extent possible.

neurodevelopmental problems, poor weight gain, learning disabilities, psychiatric disorders, and alcoholism. Thus, management of pain is a very important part of the nurse's role as a patient advocate. The margin note presents the "ABCs of Pain Management."

Patients may exhibit physical signs when they are in pain, but facial expressions and other physical responses to pain may be unique to an individual and are not valid across all patient populations. Likewise, there are no specific changes in vital signs that can be attributed solely to pain. In some cases, the patient's pulse may accelerate; in other cases, it may decelerate. Grimacing, writhing, facial tension, and guarding are some physical signs the nurse may objectively document that typically indicate the patient is experiencing discomfort.

Patients use many words to describe the pain they are experiencing; nurses should be familiar with a wide range of pain descriptors, which are presented in the margin note. No single pain assessment method or pain scale is best for all purposes. The nurse may need to use a variety of assessment techniques to evaluate fully a patient's pain status. The subjective history-gathering tool in Table 3–1 provides an organized framework to assess a patient's pain and other subjective complaints. Evaluating pain in a nonverbal pediatric or elderly patient can present unique challenges to the nurse. These patients often experience inadequate pain control by health-care providers.

EVIDENCE FOR PRACTICE: WORDS USED FOR PAIN

Aching, throbbing, shooting, stabbing, gnawing, sharp, tingling, burning, exhausting, stretching, penetrating, nagging, numb, miserable, unbearable, dull, radiating, squeezing, crampy, deep, pressure

Pain scales assist the nurse in assessing and monitoring a patient's pain level. The numeric rating scale is probably the most commonly used measure for determining a patient's pain level. In this scale, the nurse asks the patient to rate his or her pain from 0 to 10, with 0 being no pain and 10 being the worst pain. With all pain scales, the responses of the patient are valid only for that patient and that situation. A response of 5/10 in one patient will not correspond to the same report of pain in another patient. Frequent re-evaluation using the same pain scale will help the nurse *and* patient develop a consistent monitoring of the patient's pain and the response to therapeutic modalities to alleviate the pain.

In nonverbal but conscious adults, the nurse may use a visual analog scale to assess and monitor pain. In this scale, a 10-cm line is drawn with "no pain" labeled at one end and "worst pain" at the other end. The patient notes or marks his or her pain level at a corresponding point on the line.

Many pain scales have been developed for use in pediatric patients. Some of these scales use drawings or pictures of faces in pain, such as the Oucher Scale and Wong-Baker FACES Pain Rating Scale (Fig. 3–5). The Oucher Scale can include culturally appropriate pictures for assessment in patients of different races. The Poker Chip Tool asks children older than 4 years to pick the number of poker chips from a pile that corresponds to their pain level. Older children can also use numeric or visual analog scales. Pain assessment in neonates is especially challenging; the scales developed for this patient population often ask the nurse to evaluate numerous characteristics such as facial expression, sleep status, body movements, response to touch, and crying level. Nurses working with the unique populations of pediatric patients, unconscious or nonverbal adults, or patients experiencing dementia should follow the pain assessment tools recommended by their facility.

Wong-Baker FACES Pain Rating Scale

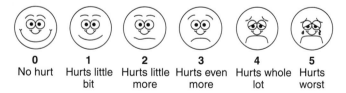

0	1	2	3	4	5
No hurt	Hurts little bit	Hurts little more	Hurts even more	Hurts whole lot	Hurts worst

Explain to the person that each face is for a person who feels happy because he has no pain (hurt) or sad because he has some or a lot of pain. Face 0 is very happy because he doesn't hurt at all. Face 2 hurts a little more. Face 3 hurts even more. Face 4 hurts a whole lot. Face 5 hurts as much as you can imagine, although you do not have to be crying to feel this bad. Ask the person to choose the face that best describes how he or she is feeling. Rating scale is recommended for persons age 3 and older.

FIGURE 3–5: FACES pain rating scale.

Chapter Summary

This chapter presented ways to master assessment, the initial step of the nursing process and a hallmark of professional practice. Use of mnemonics and reference tables will accelerate your capabilities to provide focused and systematic assessments, which contribute to desired patient outcomes and patient safety. The next chapter focuses on diagnostics, an essential part of collaborative practice.

4 Diagnostics: Understanding and Monitoring Common Laboratory Tests

CHAPTER 4

Diagnostics: Understanding and Monitoring Common Laboratory Tests

Diagnostic studies encompass a dizzying array of tests and procedures. It can be overwhelming trying to learn the important aspects of each test. Laboratory studies include analysis of blood; urine; and other patient samples such as sputum, exudates from wounds, nasal secretions, stool, and tissues. Other diagnostic tests evaluate radiological and ultrasonic views of the body, electrical rhythm of the heart (electrocardiogram [ECG]), and electrical activity of the brain (electroencephalogram [EEG]). This chapter focuses on the most commonly used laboratory diagnostic tests and basic ECG rhythms.

The nurse is often responsible for the collection and submission of samples to a facility's laboratory, initial interpretation of results, and documentation of related aspects of the nursing process. Most nurses obtain occasional experience with diagnostics during clinical rotations, practicum, and new graduate orientation, but their overall understanding remains limited because these experiences relate to orders for individual patients. As a result, many nurses feel inadequately prepared for the range of diagnostics they will encounter in daily practice. They may know to consult their facility's laboratory manual or ask department personnel when unsure about proper sample collection technique or equipment (e.g., correct blood tubes). However, many diagnostics have an element of urgency, so mastery of common diagnostics will increase confidence for everyday practice. This confidence rapidly becomes the foundation for the curiosity, commitment, and courage necessary to participate in more specialized tests and procedures.

Laboratory Test Decision Tree

During patient care, the nurse is often responsible for monitoring and reporting the results of laboratory tests for the provider. Laboratory tests (similar to drug therapy) must be reviewed within the context of the *individual patient*. Some test results may be "within normal limits" (WNL), but this result may not be the desired condition. For example, a patient at risk for blood clots (e.g., deep vein thrombosis) is often given an anticoagulant (e.g., warfarin) and then monitored with repeated international normalized ratio (INR) laboratory blood tests. In this situation, to minimize the risk of blood clots, the patient should *not* have a "normal" INR (1.0), and the provider will often seek to have an INR at a specific target greater than the normal value (e.g., 2.0 to 3.0). If the patient in this scenario had a "normal" INR, the nurse should contact the provider because of the increased risk for blood clot formation and be prepared to alter the patient's current drug therapy to achieve the desired INR.

In most patient care, however, an abnormal laboratory value is not the desired outcome, and the nurse should respond appropriately after reviewing the results of ordered laboratory tests. For some situations, established facility-generated or provider-generated protocols can guide the nurse to respond independently to abnormal laboratory test results.

- Figure 4–1 is a generic decision tree to help the nurse in working through any laboratory test result.
- Figure 4–2 is a decision tree in which the patient has an abnormally low potassium (K+) level. This decision tree identifies the subsequent steps the nurse might take and provides a model to evaluate a specific abnormal result.

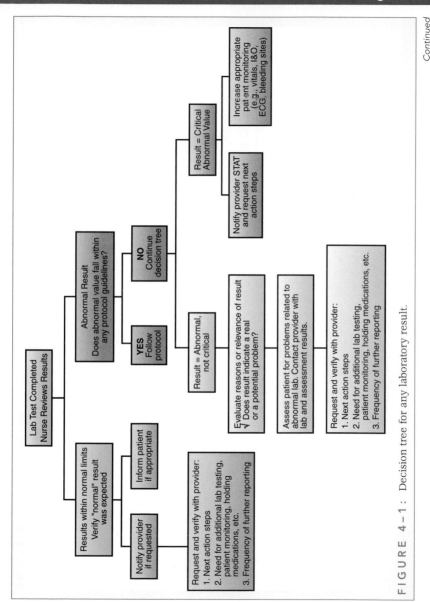

FIGURE 4–1: Decision tree for any laboratory result.

Continued

Laboratory Test Decision Tree—cont'd

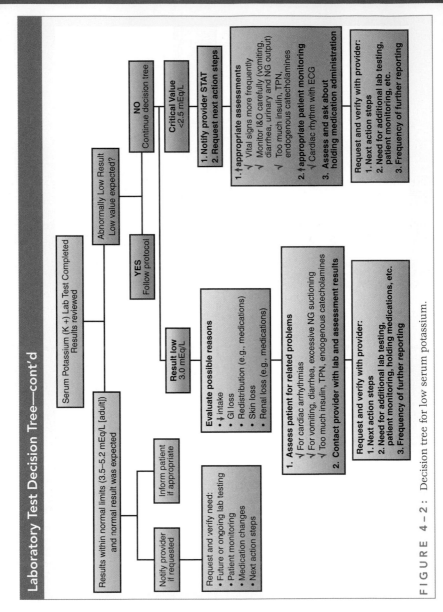

FIGURE 4–2: Decision tree for low serum potassium.

Blood Tests

Common blood diagnostic tests include the complete blood count (CBC), basic and complete metabolic panels (BMP and CMP), cardiac markers, and coagulation panels. Before reviewing the correct procedure to obtain a blood sample, review the common errors in blood collection and sampling presented in the margin notes.

Blood sampling is done most commonly through venipuncture. The nurse follows these general steps for venipuncture blood sampling:

1. Check laboratory test order (patient, time, and date). If unfamiliar with a test, check with the facility's laboratory personnel or reference manual for any special handling or transporting procedures (e.g., sample should be put on ice after venipuncture).
2. Acquire appropriate supplies: correct blood tubes, syringe or vacuumized needle and holder system (e.g., BD Vacutainer [Fig. 4–3]), tourniquet, skin cleaning and disinfecting solution, gauze, and tape or bandage.
3. Place patient in a comfortable position, and assess for latex allergies and previous venipuncture problems.
4. Wear gloves. Apply tourniquet to patient above intended venipuncture site; find and palpate an appropriate vein.

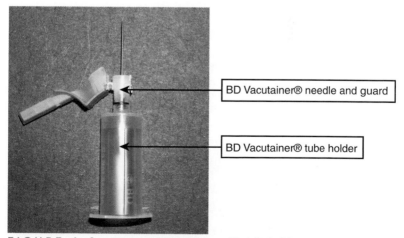

BD Vacutainer® needle and guard

BD Vacutainer® tube holder

FIGURE 4–3: BD Vacutainer system with tube holder and needle for drawing blood.

COACH CONSULT

With low values for hemoglobin and hematocrit, check for or ask for an order for a type and screen. Follow special safety procedures when collecting this blood sample, such as having a witness for the sample and verifying the patient's numbered armband. Keep current with the best evidence related to systematic criteria for type and screen (Dexter et al., 2012).

5. Clean and dry venipuncture site according to facility protocol. To prevent hemolysis and alteration of some test results, do not leave the tourniquet on for more than 1 minute before obtaining the sample.

6. Puncture skin, and obtain adequate amount of blood in correct tube order (see later). Gently invert tubes, and mix blood with additives.

7. Remove tourniquet, remove needle, and apply pressure with small gauze over puncture site. Do not have patient bend his or her elbow; this increases bleeding at the puncture site. Apply tape or bandage over gauze.

8. Document patient data, time and date, and initials of phlebotomist on each blood tube. Package blood tubes in biohazard bag, and send samples to laboratory for analysis as per facility protocol.

9. Monitor patient for problems from venipuncture.

EVIDENCE FOR PRACTICE: COMMON COLLECTION ERRORS

- Inadequate sample amount
- Inappropriate collection media or container
- Incorrect storage or temperature after collection
- Delay in delivering sample for analysis
- Incorrect or inadequate documentation on sample label

EVIDENCE FOR PRACTICE: COMMON SAMPLING ERRORS

- Blood hemolysis (needle too small, tourniquet on too long, needle bevel down, forceful draw on syringe)
- Blood drawn from above IV infusion site or not stopping infusion before draw
- Cleaning solution (alcohol) not dry before venipuncture
- Wrong order of drawing tubes
- Failure to mix (invert) blood in tube after drawing

EVIDENCE FOR PRACTICE: BLOODSTREAM INFECTIONS

Blood cultures aid in identifying the specific type of organism causing a bacterial or fungal bloodstream infection. When combined with antibiotic sensitivity tests, blood cultures provide information about which antibiotic works best against the particular organism. Contaminated samples can lead to false-positive results and inappropriate clinical interventions, which can compromise patient outcomes and incur significant expense to health-care organizations. Aseptic Non Touch Technique (ANTT) is a groundbreaking global initiative designed to improve outcomes of aseptic technique through the rationalization and standardization of practice (Rowley & Clare, 2011).

Two blood cultures taken at the time of a fever spike assist in interpreting the clinical significance of positive results and evaluating the likelihood of contamination. For example, the probability of recovering the same organism in two culture sets from a patient and of that organism being a contaminant is miniscule.

Blood cultures should be taken using a new venipuncture site and not from an existing central or peripheral venous cannula, unless it is believed that a central line may be the source of bacteremia. A peripheral vein sample should be collected first, and then blood from the central cannula should be collected. Blood cultures should not be taken from veins that are immediately proximal to an existing venous cannula. Blood cultures should not be taken from the femoral vein because it is difficult to disinfect the skin adequately, and so there is a high risk of contamination (Aziz, 2011).

When collecting multiple blood tubes, draw the blood following a specific order. In general, collect blood in tubes without additives (e.g., red top) before using tubes with additives (e.g., blue top). If unsure of the sequence of blood collection, consult your facility's laboratory manual. The Clinical and Laboratory Standards Institute recommends the following order for blood collection:

1. Blood culture tubes.
2. Waste or discard blood tubes (if necessary, use nonadditive red top).
3. Coagulation tubes (blue top) (Fig. 4–4).
4. Nonadditive tubes (red top, mottled/tiger-top serum separator tube [SST]) (see Fig. 4–4).
5. Heparin tubes (green top).
6. Ethylene diamine tetraacetic acid (EDTA) (lavender, pink, or white top) (see Fig. 4–4).
7. Oxalate-fluoride tubes (gray top).

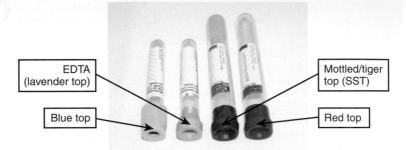

FIGURE 4-4: Common blood tubes (left to right): Coagulation tube (blue top), ethylene diamine tetraacetic acid (EDTA) (lavender top), nonadditive tubes (mottled/tiger-top SST and red top).

Tables 4–1 through 4–4 summarize what you need to know about blood collection and sampling. These tables list:
- Each test and its major components.
- The test tube or other sample collection device.
- The normal value for each component.
- Abnormal values, with possible causes for high and low values.
- Critical or panic values, if applicable.
- Nursing considerations.

The laboratory values in Tables 4–1 through 4–4 may be different from the values of an individual facility owing to a variety of diagnostic machines and standards. The values listed here for each test refer to *adults only* and appear in conventional units; many laboratories also use standard international (SI) units. The values used for these tables come from *Davis's Comprehensive Handbook of Laboratory & Diagnostic Tests With Nursing Implications* (Van Leeuwen, Poelhuis-Leth, & Bladh, 2011). Refer to this manual or consult your hospital's laboratory manual as needed and especially in the following situations:
- For abnormal values: Many drugs can alter the values of specific laboratory tests.
- For pediatric patients: Values vary significantly from infancy through childhood.

Table 4–1 lists the components of the CBC. The CBC is probably the most frequently performed blood test and has a variety of general and specific purposes.

Table 4–1 CBC*†

COMPONENT	NORMAL VALUES	ABNORMAL VALUES: POSSIBLE CAUSES		CRITICAL VALUES
		High	Low	
FREQUENTLY REVIEWED COMPONENTS				
HCT (hematocrit)	38%–44% (F) 43%–49% (M)	Dehydration, high altitude, polycythemia vera, chronic hypoxia	Anemia, alcohol abuse, hemorrhage, hemolysis, pregnancy, dilution	<18% >54%
Hgb (hemoglobin)	11.7–16.1 g/dL (F) 12.6–17.4 g/dL (M)	Dehydration, high altitude, polycythemia vera, chronic hypoxia	Anemia, alcohol abuse, hemorrhage, hemolysis, pregnancy, dilution	<6 g/dL >18 g/dL
Plt (platelet count)	150–$450 \times 10^3/mm^3$	Acute infection, anemias, heart disease, cirrhosis, liver disease, leukemias, malignancies, polycythemia vera, surgery, trauma, tuberculosis (TB)	Hemolytic anemia, disseminated intravascular coagulopathy, severe hemorrhage, leukemia, prosthetic heart valve	$<50 \times 10^3/mm^3$ $>1000 \times 10^3/mm^3$
RBC (red blood cell) count	4.2–4.87×10^3 cells/mm^3 (F) 4.71–5.14×10^3 cells/mm^3 (M)	Stress, chronic hypoxia, dehydration, high altitude, polycythemia vera, hemocon-centration	Alcohol abuse, hemolytic anemia, hemorrhage, leukemia, pregnancy, overhydration	Not applicable (N/A)

Continued

Table 4–1 CBC*†—cont'd

COMPONENT	NORMAL VALUES	ABNORMAL VALUES: POSSIBLE CAUSES		CRITICAL VALUES
		High	Low	
FREQUENTLY REVIEWED COMPONENTS—cont'd				
WBC (white blood cell) count	$4.5–11 \times 10^3$ cells/mm^3	Infections, anemias, inflammatory disorders, pregnancy, leukemias	Anemia, alcoholism, bone marrow depression, radiation, autoimmune disorders, viral infections, antineoplastic drugs	$<2.5 \times 10^3$ cells/mm^3 $>30 \times 10^3$ cells/mm^3
LESS FREQUENTLY REVIEWED COMPONENTS				
MCH (mean corpuscular hemoglobin)	28–32 pg/cell	Macrocytic anemias	Hypochromic or microcytic anemias	N/A
MCHC (mean corpuscular hemoglobin concentration)	33–35 g/dL	Macrocytic anemias	Thalassemias, spherocytosis	N/A
MCV (mean corpuscular volume)	85–95 fL	Alcoholism, liver disease, pernicious and vitamin B$_{12}$/folate anemias	Iron-deficiency anemia, thalassemias	N/A
MPV (mean platelet volume)	7.0–10.2 fL	Increased platelet turnover, leukemias, thrombocytopenic purpura, prosthetic heart valve, splenectomy, massive hemorrhage	Aplastic anemia, Wiskott-Aldrich syndrome	

Table 4–1 CBC*†—cont'd

COMPONENT	NORMAL VALUES	ABNORMAL VALUES: POSSIBLE CAUSES		CRITICAL VALUES
		High	**Low**	
LESS FREQUENTLY REVIEWED COMPONENTS—cont'd				
RDW (RBC distribution width)	11.6–14.8	Anemias	N/A	N/A

*Purpose: Basic screening of patient's blood cellular elements, RBC indices, and cell morphology.
†Nursing considerations: Fill a 5-mL lavender-top tube (EDTA) with a random blood draw. Tourniquet on <60 seconds. Avoid veins near infusing fluids. Process within 6 hours at room temperature or 24 hours refrigerated.

Table 4–2 presents the components of a basic metabolic panel (BMP) and complete metabolic panel (CMP). These tests look at the electrolyte and chemical composition of the blood. In the past, chemistry panels had other names (e.g., Chem 7, Chem 22, SMA-6, SMA-12), but more recent federal guidelines standardized the nomenclature for chemistry panels.

Table 4–3 presents blood tests related to the cardiac markers of creatine kinase myocardial band (CK-MB) fraction and cardiac troponin I and T (cTnI, cTnT). The creatine kinase test is less frequently used, and most clinicians measure serial (at 3- or 6-hour intervals) cTnI or cTnT. These tests are

(Text continues on page 124)

Table 4–2 BMP and CMP*†

COMPONENT	NORMAL VALUES	ABNORMAL VALUES: POSSIBLE CAUSES		CRITICAL VALUES
		High	**Low**	
BMP AND CMP TESTS				
Anion gap (Agap)	8–16 mEq/L	Dehydration, acidosis, poisoning, renal failure, uremia	Hypochloremia, gammaglobu-linemia, albuminemia, hyponatremia	N/A

Continued

Table 4-2 BMP and CMP*†—cont'd

COMPONENT	NORMAL VALUES	ABNORMAL VALUES: POSSIBLE CAUSES		CRITICAL VALUES
		High	Low	
		BMP AND CMP TESTS—cont'd		
Blood urea nitrogen (BUN)	8–21 mg/dL	Nephropathy, azotemia, congestive heart failure (CHF), diabetes, hyperalimentation, hypovolemia, muscle wasting, ketoacidosis	Celiac disease, malnutrition, pregnancy, liver failure	>100 mg/dL
Calcium (Ca⁺)	8.2–10.2 mg/dL	Acidosis, Addison disease, cancer, dehydration, hyperparathyroidism, Paget disease, pheochromocytoma, rhabdomyolysis, thyrotoxicosis	Alcoholism, alkalosis, chronic renal failure, pancreatitis, cirrhosis, malnutrition	<7 mg/dL >12 mg/dL
Carbon dioxide (CO_2)	22–26 mmol/L	Respiratory acidosis, metabolic alkalosis, hypoventilation, electrolyte disturbance, TB	Acute renal failure, hyperventilation, diabetic ketoacidosis, severe diarrhea, metabolic acidosis, respiratory alkalosis, salicylate poisoning	<15 mmol/L >40 mmol/L

Table 4–2 BMP and CMP*†—cont'd

COMPONENT	NORMAL VALUES	ABNORMAL VALUES: POSSIBLE CAUSES		CRITICAL VALUES
		High	**Low**	
BMP AND CMP TESTS—cont'd				
Chloride (Cl⁻)	97–107 mEq/L	Acute renal failure, Cushing syndrome, dehydration, diabetes insipidus, prolonged diarrhea, respiratory alkalosis, salicylate poisoning	Addison disease, burns, CHF, gastrointestinal (GI) loss, diabetic ketoacidosis, overhydration, respiratory acidosis	<80 mEq/L >115 mEq/L
Creatinine	0.5–1.1 mg/dL (F) 0.6–1.2 mg/dL (M)	CHF, dehydration, rhabdomyolysis, shock, hyperthyroidism, renal failure	Inadequate protein intake, pregnancy, liver disease	>7.4 mg/dL
Glucose (blood sugar)	65–99 mg/dL (fasting)	Acute stress, trauma, diabetes, hemochromatosis, myocardial infarction (MI), pancreatitis, strenuous exercise, thyrotoxicosis	Alcohol ingestion, Addison disease, hypothyroidism, glycogen storage diseases, starvation, excess insulin	<40 mg/dL >400 mg/dL
Potassium (K⁺)	3.5–5 mEq/L	Acidosis, diabetes, renal failure, increased intake, dehydration, hemolysis, ketoacidosis, tissue trauma, pregnancy	Alcoholism, inadequate intake, Cushing syndrome, excess insulin, gastrointestinal loss, pica	<2.5 mEq/L >6.5 mEq/L

Continued

Table 4-2 BMP and CMP*†—cont'd

COMPONENT	NORMAL VALUES	ABNORMAL VALUES: POSSIBLE CAUSES		CRITICAL VALUES
		High	Low	
BMP AND CMP TESTS—cont'd				
Sodium (Na+)	135–145 mEq/L	Azotemia, dehydration, Cushing syndrome, excessive intake, vomiting	Addison disease, CHF, cirrhosis, cystic fibrosis, excessive diuretics, inadequate intake, renal failure, syndrome of inappropriate diuretic hormone (SIADH), water intoxication	<120 mEq/L >160 mEq/L
CMP TESTS ONLY				
Albumin (Alb)	3.4–4.8 g/dL	Dehydration, blood loss	Malabsorption, malnutrition, liver disease, infection, burns, pregnancy, nephropathy	N/A
Alkaline phosphatase (ALP)	25–125 U/L (F) 35–142 U/L (M)	Liver disease, bone disease, pregnancy, atherosclerosis	Anemia, celiac disease, nutritional deficiencies	N/A
Alanine aminotransferase (ALT), serum glutamic pyruvic transaminase (SGPT)	7–35 U/L (F) 10–40 U/L (M)	Acute pancreatitis, alcohol abuse, cirrhosis, traumatic muscle injury, hepatitis, mononucleosis, shock	Pyridoxal phosphate deficiency	N/A

Table 4–2 BMP and CMP*†—cont'd

COMPONENT	NORMAL VALUES	ABNORMAL VALUES: POSSIBLE CAUSES		CRITICAL VALUES
		High	Low	
CMP TESTS ONLY—cont'd				
Aspartate aminotransferase (AST), serum glutamic oxaloacetic transaminase (SGOT)	9–36 U/L (F) 19–48 U/L (M)	Hepatitis, pancreatitis, shock, biliary obstruction, hemolytic anemia, CHF, muscle damage	N/A	N/A
Bilirubin, total (Tbil)	0.3–1.2 mg/dL	Hepatic jaundice, cirrhosis, hepatitis, mononucleosis, pernicious anemia, anorexia/starvation	N/A	>15 mg/dL
Phosphorus (phosphate [PO$_4$])	2.5–4.5 mg/dL	Acromegaly, bone diseases, renal failure, diabetic ketoacidosis, respiratory acidosis, hypocalcemia	Hypercalcemia, hyperparathyroidism, hypokalemia, gout, severe vomiting/diarrhea, respiratory alkalosis	<1 mg/dL N/A
Protein, total (TP)	6–8 g/dL	Dehydration, myeloma, sarcoidosis	Burns, blood loss, malnutrition, malabsorption, nephritic syndrome, pregnancy, prolonged immobilization	

*Purpose: Evaluation of various chemical blood constituents, especially electrolytes, blood urea nitrogen (BUN), and glucose.

†Nursing considerations: Fill (~5 mL) and invert a red- or marbled (tiger)-top tube with a random, timed, or fasting blood draw. Avoid veins near infusing fluids. Process promptly. Try to keep tourniquet on <60 seconds; a tourniquet on for a long time can cause venous stasis and hemolysis, which can affect some chemistry tests.

Table 4–3 Cardiac Markers

TEST	NORMAL VALUES	ABNORMAL RESULTS: POSSIBLE CAUSES OF HIGH VALUES ONLY
Creatine kinase myocardial band (CK-MB)	<4%–6% (electrophoresis) <10 ng/mL (immunoassay)	MI, cerebrovascular accident (CVA), pericarditis, rhabdomyolysis, cardiomyopathy, cardioversion *Critical value: N/A*
Troponin I (cTnI)	<0.35 ng/mL	Small infarcts, myocardial damage post cardiac surgery *Critical value: >1.5 ng/mL*
Troponin T (cTnT)	<0.20 ng/mL	Acute MI, myocardial damage post cardiac surgery or angioplasty, unstable angina, myocarditis, trauma, rhabdomyolysis *Critical value: N/A*

generally used to evaluate possible heart muscle damage in conditions such as suspected acute myocardial infarction (MI) and myocardial ischemia.

Table 4–4 lists the components of coagulation panels and includes the individual tests of prothrombin time (PT), from which the international normalized ratio (INR), activated partial thromboplastin time (APTT), and D-dimer are derived. Because PT and INR evaluate the ability of blood to clot properly, they can be used to assess bleeding and clotting tendencies. One common use of these tests is to monitor the effectiveness of anticoagulant drugs, such as warfarin (Coumadin).

Urinalysis

For patient urine samples, urinalysis (UA) is a frequently used diagnostic test. Culturing a patient's urine is also a common diagnostic test. Table 4–5 shows the components of the frequently run UA. UA most commonly requires a clean-catch technique. The nurse explains the following steps to a male or female patient:

Male:

1. Have patient wash hands thoroughly.
2. Have patient cleanse the penile meatus from the center outward by using a washcloth with soap and water or urine sample collection kit cleansing towelettes (Peri-Wipes).

Table 4–4 Coagulation Panels*†

TEST	NORMAL VALUES	ABNORMAL VALUES: POSSIBLE CAUSES		CRITICAL VALUES
		High	**Low**	
PT **INR**	10–13 sec <2.0	Disseminated intravascular coagulation (DIC), hereditary factor (II, V, VII, X) disorders, cirrhosis, decreased fat absorption, causes of vitamin K deficiency, excess anticoagulant	Ovarian hyperfunction, enteritis, or ileitis	>3.0
APTT	25–39 sec	DIC, hemophilia factor deficiencies, polycythemia, severe liver disease, vitamin K deficiency, von Willebrand disease, excess heparin	N/A	>60 sec
D-Dimer	No detectable fragments (semiquantitative) <250 ng/mL (quantitative)	Arterial or venous thrombosis, deep vein thrombosis (DVT), DIC, neoplastic disease, pre-eclampsia, pregnancy, pulmonary embolism (PE), recent surgery (within 2 days), secondary fibrinolysis, thrombolytic or fibrinolytic therapy	N/A	N/A

*Purpose: All tests are used in some way to evaluate coagulation. PT/INR is used specifically to monitor warfarin therapy. The INR is derived from the PT value and is used to normalize ratios across different laboratories. APTT is used specifically to monitor heparin therapy. D-dimer is used specifically to help detect DIC, DVT, MI, and PE.

†Nursing considerations: Completely fill (~5 mL) and invert blue-top (sodium citrate) tube with a random or timed blood draw. Partially filled tubes cannot be analyzed. Do not draw coagulation blood tests from a heparinized catheter. Keep tourniquet on <60 seconds; a tourniquet on for a long time can cause venous stasis and hemolysis, which can affect tests.

Table 4–5 **UA***†			
TEST	**NORMAL VALUES**	**ABNORMAL RESULTS: POSSIBLE CAUSES OF HIGH VALUES ONLY**	
		High	**Low**
Color	Pale yellow (straw-colored) to amber	Dark yellow may indicate dehydration; drugs, food, or metabolic by-products may alter urine color	Colorless urine may indicate overhydration
Appearance	Clear to slightly hazy	Cloudy urine may be due to pus, RBCs, bacteria, semen, vaginal discharges, or ingestion of certain foods or supplements	N/A
Specific gravity	1.005–1.030	CHF, dehydration, diabetes, nephritic syndrome, SIADH	Chronic renal failure, diabetes insipidus, glomerulonephritis
pH	5–9	Citrus fruits, alkalosis, vegetarian diet	High-protein ingestion, fruits (cranberries), acidosis
Protein	<20 mg/dL	Diabetic nephropathy, glomerulonephritis, toxemia of pregnancy, stress, exercise	N/A
Glucose	Negative	Diabetes, Cushing syndrome, acromegaly	N/A
Ketones	Negative	Acute illness, diabetes, diabetic ketoacidosis (DKA), fasting, high-protein diet, postanesthesia vomiting, strenuous exercise	N/A
Hemoglobin	Negative	Renal calculi/trauma, malignancy, urinary tract infection (UTI), glomerulonephritis, systemic hemolysis, polycystic kidney disease, menstruation	N/A

Table 4–5 UA*†—cont'd

TEST	NORMAL VALUES	ABNORMAL RESULTS: POSSIBLE CAUSES OF HIGH VALUES ONLY	
		High	**Low**
Bilirubin	Negative	Cirrhosis, hepatitis, hepatic tumor, obstructive biliary disease	N/A
Urobilinogen	<1 mg/dL	Cirrhosis, hepatitis, CHF, hemolytic anemia, mononucleosis, pernicious anemia, malaria	N/A
Nitrite	Negative	Nitrite-forming bacteria, UTI	N/A
Leukocyte esterase	Negative	Bacterial, fungal, or parasitic infection; glomerulonephritis; nephritis	N/A

*Purpose: Evaluate various constituents of patient's urine for screening and diagnostic purposes. Urine may also be cultured to screen for bacterial infection.

†Nursing considerations: Generally, a random, clean sample of ~30 mL is obtained from either a "clean-catch" (see text) or from the drainage bag of an indwelling catheter. A clean urine collection cup is typically used to send the sample to the laboratory, but a sterile red-top tube can also be used. In a few urine tests, a "dirty" urine sample is collected. Nurses sometimes do a unit-based "dipstick" urinalysis, which uses biochemical markers on a small stick dipped into the urine to provide information for diagnostic purposes. Urine is usually tested at room temperature. Urine should be refrigerated if a delay in transport to the laboratory is expected.

3. Have patient void a small amount of urine into the toilet. (A few urine tests require a urine sample that is not clean-catch. The patient should collect urine from the initial voiding.)
4. Have patient void "midstream" urine into collection cup.
5. The patient should replace lid on collection cup and give urine sample to the nurse to record date, time, and initials and send to laboratory for analysis.

Female:
1. Have patient wash hands thoroughly.
2. Have patient spread and cleanse the labia from front to back by using a washcloth with soap and water or urine sample collection kit towelettes (Peri-Wipes).

3. While keeping labia open, have patient void a small amount of urine into the toilet. Without stopping the urine stream, have patient void into collection cup.

🗣 CLINICAL VOICE: A MOST UNUSUAL DIAGNOSTIC TEST

Our vicarious nursing instructor and mentor Dr. Laura Gasparis Vonfrolio tells a remarkable story of discovering hyperglycemic hyperosmolar nonketosis (HHNK) in Mary, a resident at a long-term care facility. As Dr. Vonfrolio walked through Mary's room, she stepped in a puddle of an obviously sticky solution. She asked what might be on the floor, and Mary replied, "Oh, I was feeling rather tired and 'passed water' when I couldn't get to the bathroom quickly." Dr. Vonfrolio realized the syrupy solution could be due to a severely elevated blood glucose level and took quick action to have Mary transported to a hospital, where laboratory reports soon confirmed a blood glucose level greater than 900 mg/dL. In HHNK, symptoms can include weakness, increased thirst, nausea, lethargy, confusion, and, ultimately, convulsions and coma. Onset of these symptoms can be slow and insidious, building over days or weeks. Mary received appropriate treatment and soon returned to her facility.

ALERT

Many respiratory illnesses do not give a high Paco$_2$ result on arterial blood gases (ABGs) unless the patient is close to death. With respiratory diseases, a decrease in Paco$_2$ is the first sign of impending respiratory failure. A decrease in Paco$_2$ with no change in Pao$_2$ means the patient is very sick, and the nurse must notify the physician with that critical message.

Interpreting Arterial Blood Gases

Arterial blood gases (ABGs) refer to any of the gases present in blood. Clinically, they include the determination of levels of pH, oxygen, and carbon dioxide in the blood. ABGs are important in the diagnosis and treatment of disturbances of:

- Acid-base balance.
- Pulmonary disease.
- Electrolyte balance.
- Oxygen delivery.

Patients with respiratory, cardiac, renal, and metabolic disorders have ABG samples taken, often in emergent situations. Understanding ABG results is an essential part of patient care, making patient assessment more informed and patient management more specific. ABG interpretation confounds many nurses, yet mastery of this particular skill makes a nurse better prepared not only as a patient advocate but also as a valued resource for team members and even other units, especially at 3 a.m.!

Common approaches to ABG interpretation include a six-step analysis, a three-step analysis, and arrow-up/arrow-down using the ROME mnemonic (Respiratory Opposite, Metabolic Equal). In our experience, students cannot learn or retain ABG interpretation through these approaches. Instead, we endorse Vonfrolio's systematic number-line method, which consists of two steps. In this section, we walk you through the two steps, guide you through practice examples, and give you ABGs to interpret on your own with the answers immediately following.

COACH CONSULT

Without fail, of more than 40 students in a section of senior practicum, only 2 can interpret ABGs, typically because they already work in an emergency department. We offer a two-step method as taught by nurse educator Laura Gasparis Vonfrolio, PhD, RN, CEN, CCRN. At the end of a 40-minute session, all our students can interpret ABGs.

Two-Step Approach to ABG Interpretation
Step 1: Look at the pH
- To obtain the first and last name of the imbalance, place the pH value on the number line.

Step 2: Look at Paco$_2$ and HCO$_3^-$
- To obtain the middle name of the imbalance, determine whether Paco$_2$ or HCO$_3^-$ has the same last name according to placement on the number line.

First Name Choices:	Middle Name Choices (can be both):	Last Name Choices:
Uncompensated	Respiratory	Acidosis
Compensated	Metabolic	Alkalosis

Number-Line Evaluation of ABG Values

Normal Ranges

pH

Uncompensated Acidosis   < 7.35–7.45 >   Uncompensated Alkalosis

Paco$_2$

(Respiratory Acid)

Respiratory Alkalosis   < 35–45 >   Respiratory Acidosis

$$HCO_3^-$$
(Metabolic Base)

Metabolic Acidosis   < 22–26 >   Metabolic Alkalosis

Compensated Gases

Compensated Acidosis 7.35   < 7.40 >   7.45 Compensated Alkalosis

Step 1: Practice

1. If pH is 7.12, the first name is uncompensated; the last name is acidosis.
2. If pH is 7.55, the first name is uncompensated; the last name is alkalosis.
3. If pH is 7.02, the first name is uncompensated; the last name is acidosis.
4. If pH is 7.60, the first name is uncompensated; the last name is alkalosis

You try a couple, which are typical values in NCLEX-RN scenarios:

5. If pH is 7.48, the first name is _____; the last name is _____.
6. If pH is 7.30, the first name is _____; the last name is _____.

In Question 5, the first name is uncompensated, the last name is alkalosis.
In Question 6, the first name is uncompensated, the last name is acidosis.
So that's easy! Now, add the second step.

Steps 1–2: Practice

ABG results: pH 7.21, Paco$_2$ 32, HCO$_3^-$ 14

1. If pH is 7.21, the first name is uncompensated; the last name is acidosis.
2. What has the same last name?
   Does a Paco$_2$ of 32 indicate acidosis? *No*
   Does an HCO$_3^-$ of 14 indicate metabolic acidosis? *Yes*
   Result: Uncompensated metabolic acidosis.

ABG results: pH 7.18, Paco$_2$ 68, HCO$_3^-$ 29

1. If pH is 7.18, the first name is uncompensated; the last name is acidosis.
2. What has the same last name?
   Does a Paco$_2$ of 68 indicate acidosis? *Yes*
   Does an HCO$_3^-$ of 29 indicate metabolic acidosis? *No*
   Result: Uncompensated respiratory acidosis

ABG results: pH 7.50, Paco$_2$ 26, HCO$_3^-$ 21

1. If pH is 7.50, the first name is uncompensated; the last name is alkalosis.

2. What has the same last name?
Does a Paco$_2$ of 26 indicate alkalosis? *Yes*
Does an HCO$_3^-$ of 21 indicate alkalosis? *No*
Result: Uncompensated respiratory alkalosis

ABG results: pH 7.52, Paco$_2$ 36, HCO$_3^-$ 34

1. If pH is 7.52, the first name is uncompensated; the last name is alkalosis.
2. What has the same last name?
Does a Paco$_2$ of 36 indicate alkalosis? *No*
Does an HCO$_3^-$ of 34 indicate alkalosis? *Yes*
Result: Uncompensated metabolic alkalosis

ABG results: pH 7.36, Paco$_2$ 54, HCO$_3^-$ 32

1. If pH is 7.36, the first name is compensated; the last name is acidosis.
2. What has the same last name?
Does a Paco$_2$ of 54 indicate acidosis? *Yes*
Does an HCO$_3^-$ of 32 indicate acidosis? *No*
Result: Compensated respiratory acidosis

Common ABG Profiles

Accelerate your mastery of ABG interpretation by having possible scenarios or a mental picture of a patient for each common acid-base disturbance. If you see a patient with a chronic obstructive pulmonary disease (COPD) exacerbation, for example, predict the ABG result. You will tune up your critical thinking skills simultaneously. Following are profiles of the four most common acid-base disturbances.

Uncompensated Respiratory Acidosis
Sample ABG: pH 7.18, Paco$_2$ 68, HCO$_3^-$ 29
Possible causes:

- Hypoventilation (COPD exacerbation)
- Wrong medications (e.g., gentamicin given to a patient with myasthenia gravis, which precipitates a myasthenic crisis—the patient develops ptosis and dysphagia and drools; then a decreased respiratory rate leads to a decreased tidal volume and a respiratory arrest)
- Too much of some medications (e.g., opioid narcotics such as morphine sulfate)

Notes:

- Sodium bicarbonate (HCO$_3^-$, bicarb) is *not* recommended for respiratory acidosis unless the patient is intubated and needs medications that will not work in an acidotic environment, such as some medications for patients with asthma. Do you know why? Sodium bicarbonate increases CO_2 production: $HCO_3^- + H^+$ (other acids) $\rightarrow H_2CO_3$ (carbonic acid) $\rightarrow H_2O + CO_2$ ($\uparrow$ respiratory acid, an excess of which caused the disturbance).

Uncompensated Metabolic Acidosis
Sample ABG: pH 7.21, Paco$_2$ 32, HCO$_3^-$ 14

Possible causes:

- Renal failure, because patients do not excrete all their sulfuric and phosphoric acids
- Diabetic ketoacidosis
- Low blood pressure, which leads to vasoconstriction, which deprives muscles of blood supply, which causes a buildup in lactic acid

Notes:

When the pH falls below 7.25, the blood vessels vasodilate, and the patient becomes mottled from pooling of blood in the capillaries. The low blood pressure becomes lower from tachycardia, and the patient goes into shock.

Treatment is isotonic fluids (or hypertonic fluids if the patient is postoperative) and possibly sodium bicarbonate if the physician believes the acidosis will not correct quickly.

Uncompensated Respiratory Alkalosis
Sample ABG: pH 7.50, Paco$_2$ 26, HCO$_3^-$ 21

Possible causes:

- Anxiety or panic attack
- Pain (MI)
- Cirrhosis (elevated ammonia [NH$_3$] levels, which make the medulla increase the respiratory rate to 28 to 32 breaths per minute)

Notes:

Correct alkalosis because:

- Alkalosis causes calcium to go into cells: low serum Ca^{++} causes numbness and tingling (watch for Chvostek and Trousseau signs).
- Alkalosis causes a shift in the oxyhemoglobin dissociation curve: A pulse oximeter may show adequate oxygen saturation, but less

oxygen is let off to the tissues. For example, a patient with MI has anxiety and pain, which increase the respiratory rate. Less oxygen is let off to ischemic tissues, which could extend an infarct. In addition to aspirin and nitroglycerin, expect to give morphine sulfate and oxygen.

Uncompensated Metabolic Alkalosis

Sample ABG: pH 7.52, $Paco_2$ 36, HCO_3^- 34

Possible causes:

- Nasogastric tube to suction
- Too much lactated Ringer solution (lactate is converted to sodium bicarbonate by a functioning liver)

Notes:

- Treatment requires hospital therapy and monitoring: Sodium chloride (NaCl) is given because in alkalosis, H^+ comes out of the cell into the serum. However, the kidneys, in response to the increased acidosis, increase production of sodium bicarbonate, which worsens the condition. The remedy is to flood the kidneys with NaCl, which will dissociate. The kidneys will not hold onto an excess of negatively charged sodium bicarbonate when bombarded with another negative ion (Cl^-).

EVIDENCE FOR PRACTICE: OXYGEN COLLECTION

Remember the oxygen (Pao_2)! ABGs also provide critical information about a patient's oxygen delivery. If the Pao_2 level is low, immediately check for a mechanical problem. Is the oxygen connected with correct liter flow? Next, consider what the patient's Pao_2 level is supposed to be. Take the percentage of oxygen your patient is receiving and multiply by 6 (the formula constant). Subtract the $Paco_2$. Subtract the Pao_2. Example: A patient is on 30% O_2 by face mask. His ABG results show a pH of 7.35 (normal), Pao_2 of 70, and $Paco_2$ of 45 (normal). Calculate: $30 \times 6 = 180 - 45 = 135$. The Pao_2 is supposed to be 135, but it is only 70. The difference ($135 - 70 = 65$) is called an oxygen delivery gradient. A patient is not supposed to have a gradient (the difference is supposed to be close to 0), so there is a problem with his oxygen delivery (as a result of atelectasis, pneumonia, pulmonary edema, acute respiratory distress syndrome [ARDS], or another pulmonary disease process).

Interpreting Electrocardiograms

Although electrocardiogram (ECG) interpretation receives more attention in telemetry units and critical care areas, for patient safety every nurse must know how to read and interpret basic rhythms. Table 4–6, "Fast Facts for a Comprehensive ECG Assessment," presents a comprehensive overview.

Table 4–6 Fast Facts for a Comprehensive ECG Assessment

CARDIAC CELLS	PROPERTIES	
Electrical cells	Automaticity: Cell's ability to generate and discharge an electrical impulse spontaneously Excitability: Cell's ability to transmit an electrical impulse Conductivity: Cell's ability to transmit an electrical impulse from one cell to another	
Myocardial cells	Contractility: Ability of cell filaments to shorten and return to their original shape Extensibility: Ability of cell filaments to stretch	
ELECTRICAL CONDUCTION SYSTEM	PACEMAKER CELLS	SEEN AS:
Sinoatrial (SA) node	Fire at 60–100 times/min	P wave: Atrial depolarization (impulse through SA node)
Internodal tracts Interatrial tracts (Bachmann bundle)		P-R interval: Time required to leave SA and travel to AV node, bundle of His, bundle branches, and Purkinje fibers
Atrioventricular	Fire at 40–60 times/min (AV) node	
Bundle of His		
Right and left bundle branches		
Purkinje fibers, ventricular node	Fire at 20–30 times/min	QRS ventricular depolarization (impulse through ventricles)

Table 4–6 **Fast Facts for a Comprehensive ECG Assessment—cont'd**

CARDIAC CYCLE	PROPERTIES	NORMAL (Fig. 4–5)
P wave	Atrial depolarization (impulse through SA node)	Small, rounded, positive (upright) in lead II with amplitude 0.5–2.5 mm, duration 0.10 sec or less
PR interval	Time required to leave SA node and travel through AV node to bundle of His and bundle branches to Purkinje fibers	From beginning P to beginning of QRS: 0.12–0.20 sec
QRS complex	Ventricular depolarization (impulse through ventricles)	Beginning of QRS to ST segment: amplitude 2–15 mm and 0.04–0.10 sec
ST segment	End of ventricular depolarization and beginning of repolarization	End of QRS to onset of T wave, normally flat (isoelectric) or follows the isometric line Abnormal: Elevation/depression by 1 mm or more above/below baseline or 0.08 sec or 2 small squares past J point

F I G U R E   4 – 5 :   Normal ECG tracing with identified parts.

Continued

Table 4–6 Fast Facts for a Comprehensive ECG Assessment—cont'd

CARDIAC CYCLE	PROPERTIES	NORMAL (see Fig. 4–5)
T wave	Latter phase of ventricular depolarization	Rounded, asymmetrical (peak closer to end of the wave than the beginning) positive in lead II with an amplitude less than 5 mm
Refractory period divided into: Absolute refractory period Relative refractory period	Time during cardiac cycle when cardiac cells may or may not be depolarized by an electrical stimulus (depends on strength of impulse) From QRS to peak of T wave: Cardiac cells have not repolarized to their threshold; cannot be stimulated to depolarize (electrical cells cannot conduct impulse, and myocardial cells cannot contract) Begins at peak of T wave to end of T wave: Cardiac cells have repolarized sufficiently to respond to a strong stimulus (e.g., PVC contraction)	
Q-T interval	Time between onset of ventricular depolarization and end of ventricular repolarization	From beginning of QRS complex to end of T wave; normal is corrected for heart rate but usually less than half of R-R interval
U wave	Further repolarization	Small, rounded; <2 mm in height and deflection is same as T wave
ECG	PROPERTIES	
ECG	Propagation of electrical impulses from cell to cell produces an electrical current, which can be detected by skin electrodes and recorded as waves or deflections on graph paper	
Lead	A monitor lead provides a view of the heart's electrical activity between two points or poles (positive and negative) Direction of current flow: Direction of wave form Toward positive pole: Positive deflection Toward negative pole: Negative deflection Perpendicular to pole: Positive and negative deflection	

Table 4–6 Fast Facts for a Comprehensive ECG Assessment—cont'd

ECG	PROPERTIES
Paper	Horizontal lines: Duration of waveforms in seconds of time (each small square = 0.04 sec) (each small square measured vertically = 1 mm in height) Vertical lines: Voltage or amplitude of waveforms in mm

ANALYSIS OF RHYTHM STRIP	PROCEDURE
Determine regularity or rhythm of R waves	Measure R wave to R wave across strip Variation of 0.12 sec in R-wave regularity = irregular rhythm
Calculate heart rate	Regular rhythms: Equal distance on all R-R intervals Rapid rate calculation: Count number of R waves in a 6-second strip and multiply by 10 = heart rate per minute Precise rate calculation: Count number of small squares between two consecutive R waves and use conversion chart (300, 150, 100, 75, 60, 50, 43, 38, 33, 30, 27, 25, 23, 21, 19, 18, 16) or divide number of small squares between two consecutive R waves into 1500
Identify and examine P waves	One P wave should precede each QRS complex, and all should be identical (or near identical) in size, shape, and position
Measure P-R interval	Measure from beginning of P wave as it leaves baseline to beginning of QRS complex
Measure QRS complex	Measure from beginning of QRS as it leaves baseline until end of QRS when ST segment begins
Based on above analysis, interpret rhythm	Interpret rhythm
ECG interpretation Summary	Rate: Measure with rapid rate or precise rate calculation Rhythm: P before QRS; P-R interval, QRS interval; measure R-R with calipers Axis: QRS above or below baseline Hypertrophy: V1—Check P wave, R wave, S wave for various areas Infarction: Check all leads for Q waves, inverted T waves, ST segment depression or elevation

Created by Dana D. Daughtry, BSN RN; adapted from Huff, J. (2012). *ECG workout: Exercises in arrhythmia interpretation* (6th ed.). Ambler, PA: Lippincott, Williams & Wilkins.

We recommend evaluation of six aspects of a rhythm strip:

1. Rate.
2. Rhythm.
3. Complete/abnormal complexes.
4. Axis.
5. Hypertrophy.
6. Infarction.

Let's look at each of the six aspects in more detail:

1. Rate:
   - Check patient's pulse (apical and radial for perfusion in abnormal rhythms such as atrial fibrillation).
   - Start at large box bold line that coincides with an R wave.
   - Count down: 300, 150, 100, 75, 60, 50 at each large box bold line until you come to the next R wave.
   - If the R wave is between two large box lines, use Table 4–7, "Calculating Heart Rate," to determine the exact rate.
   - For bradycardia, the rate = number of complexes/6-second strip × 10.

Table 4–7 **Calculating Heart Rate***

NUMBER OF LARGE BOXES	RATE/MIN	NUMBER OF SMALL BOXES	RATE/MIN
1	300	2	750
2	150	3	500
3	100	4	375
4	75	5	300
5	60	6	250
6	50	7	214
7	43	8	186
8	38	9	167
9	33	10	150
10	30	11	136

Table 4-7 Calculating Heart Rate*—cont'd

NUMBER OF LARGE BOXES	RATE/MIN	NUMBER OF SMALL BOXES	RATE/MIN
11	27	12	125
12	25	13	115
13	23	14	107
14	21	15	100
15	20	16	94

*Clinical tip: Approximate rate per minute is rounded to the next highest number.

From Jones, S. A. (2009). *ECG notes: Interpretation and management guide* (2nd ed.). Philadelphia, PA: F. A. Davis.

2. Rhythm:
   - Use calipers to measure distance between two consecutive R waves; measure distance between the next R waves; the distance is equal in a regular rhythm and unequal in an irregular rhythm.
   - Sinus rhythm = regular rhythm and rate 60 to 100 bpm and regular.
   - Sinus tachycardia = regular rhythm and rate greater than 100 bpm.
   - Sinus bradycardia = regular rhythm and rate less than 60 bpm.
   - Sinus arrhythmia = varies with respiratory phase.
   - Atrial fibrillation = irregular ventricular rhythm with no P waves.
   - Sinoatrial (SA) node dysfunction = sinus block, sick sinus syndrome.
   - Premature beats = premature atrial contractions (PACs), premature ventricular contractions (PVCs).
   - Tachyarrhythmias = PACs, PVCs; flutter, fibrillation.
   - Sinus blocks = AV blocks (indicated by abnormal P-R interval), bundle branch block (indicated by abnormal QRS interval), hemiblock (indicated by pathologic axis deviation).
   - Dissociated rhythms = independent atrial and ventricular rates.

3. Complete/abnormal complexes:
   - For each complex, is there a P wave?
   - For each complex, is there a QRS wave?
   - Flat P wave.
   - Long P-R interval.
   - F or f waves.
   - Wide QRS complex.
4. Axis (electrical):
   - Check if QRS complex is positive or negative in lead I and AVF (up in lead I and AVF = normal; down in lead I and AVF = bad).
5. Hypertrophy:
   - Check V1 lead (P wave for atrial hypertrophy, R wave for right ventricular hypertrophy, S-wave depth, positive R-wave height in V5 for left ventricular hypertrophy).
6. Infarction:
   - Presence of Q wave = necrosis.
   - ST segment elevation = injury, acute (with Q waves = acute, recent infarct).
   - ST segment depression that persists = subendocardial infarction.
   - T-wave inversion = ischemia (often found with Q-wave or ST segment elevation).
   - Compare with previous ECGs if available.

Chapter Summary

This chapter presented common diagnostics that are critical to your competent practice. Nurses play a vital role on the interprofessional team related to diagnostics, including collection and submission of samples to a facility's laboratory, initial interpretation of results, and documentation of related aspects of the nursing process. We hope you feel better prepared from reading this chapter for the range of diagnostics you will encounter in daily practice, whether they are urgent or routine. The next chapter presents key features of patient care. The content emphasizes critical skills, patient safety, and management of machines.

5 Patient Care: Reviewing Critical Skills, Keeping Patients Safe, and Managing Machines

Patient Care: Reviewing Critical Skills, Keeping Patients Safe, and Managing Machines

In Chapter 1, we provided a list of basic nursing skills, grouped according to the nursing process, that a generalist nurse should be comfortable performing after completing nursing school. This chapter is an overview of selected critical skills that nurses perform. With the emphasis on quality and safety in nursing, particularly driven by the QSEN Institute, competence in these skills is expected, but becoming expert in performing any nursing skill requires time and experience. Therefore, for these skills we provide a detailed review with expert tips to accelerate your mastery. Ultimately, your own repetition, refinement, and reflection on safe, evidence-based practice contribute more in the development of skill expertise.

Beginning in Chapter 1 we emphasized that the nursing process is applicable in all care settings and to all patient populations. We also noted that the steps of the nursing process follow the mnemonic ADOPIE. Nurses habitually begin their patient care with a relevant Assessment. Using critical thinking and clinical judgment, they develop a nursing Diagnosis and identify Outcomes that guide their path to the desired end. With this perspective, they Plan and Implement targeted interventions. After they initiate any therapeutic intervention, nurses Evaluate their actions and the patient's response. The cycle of the nursing process continues with re-Assessment.

COACH CONSULT

Nursing's innovative leaders in caring science include Marian C. Turkel and Marilyn Ann Ray. They propose renaming the nursing process based on nursing's language of caring. Their mnemonic RCPR (think: "relational CPR") stands for *Recognizing, Connecting, Partnering,* and *Reflecting.*

One of the nurse's main activities in patient care is to provide or supervise therapeutic interventions using nursing skills. Nursing skills are often the "hands-on" part of nursing care, but these technical skills are not all that a nurse does. Critical analysis of clinical situations may be invisible, but it is the foundation for safe and effective nursing skills.

In a research study, senior nursing students cited nine skills, listed subsequently, with which they needed more help and repetition to be ready for professional nursing practice. In our experience, newly practicing nurses and their preceptors also need more guidance with these skills. Therefore, for each skill, we review the procedure and add comments to emphasize quality, safety, or other important considerations. For all skills, refer to specific facility protocols as well.

- Starting an IV infusion
- Inserting a nasogastric tube (NGT)
- Inserting an indwelling (Foley) urinary catheter
- Administering a blood transfusion
- Mixing two types of insulin
- Performing tracheostomy care
- Taking orthostatic vital signs
- Performing an electrocardiogram (ECG)
- Managing basic bedside monitoring

Starting an IV Infusion

Although starting an IV infusion is a common nursing intervention, it has many important aspects that relate directly to patient safety. *Manual of I.V. Therapeutics,* published by F.A. Davis and authored by a recent past president of the Infusion Nurses Society (INS), comprehensively covers these elements of safe, evidence-based infusion therapy (Phillips, 2010). IV infusions may be used for various fluids, medications, or diagnostic solutions (dye). An IV tube is a direct external connection to the internal circulatory system; proper insertion, maintenance, and monitoring are important to protect patients from infection. It is critical to administer medications correctly through an IV line because the drug quickly disperses through the circulatory system. Starting IV lines on pediatric patients requires special training; in contrast to in adults, sites in the scalp, leg, or feet are often used. Table 5–1, "Starting an IV Infusion," outlines the steps used for a typical IV insertion in an adult.

CLINICAL VOICE: FINELY HONED NURSING SKILLS

It was still early into the beginning of another night shift when the child arrived at the triage area of our community hospital's ER. He was being carried by his father. The mother was hovering close by. The parents were very anxious and the child was listless and lethargic. They were from Vietnam and their English was minimal, adding to our difficulty in finding out what was going on. The child was moved immediately to our critical care room.

The 4-year-old had been sick for the past 4 days with vomiting, diarrhea, and fever. The parents had tried to treat their son as best they could; however, the child continued to get worse. He was lethargic, pale, non-responsive, and flaccid. I immediately called the ER physician and started setting up for an IV. Starting an IV is a routine I've done a thousand times, and it sometimes seems the basic nursing skills we do every day are just practice for the one time it will really make a difference. As the physician entered the room he recognized the severity of the child's condition and after my first attempt at inserting an IV failed, he tried to find access. Two IO attempts and two punctures left us still without any access. I can remember the intense focus I had as I looked at the hand of the child and knew I could "get a line in." A few moments later and we were pushing fluid through the IV tubing in the child's hand and breathing a big sigh of relief that we could now revive the child.

Soon, the pediatrician on-call arrived and arranged for transport of the child to the children's hospital in a nearby city where I also worked part-time in the ER. By calling to their ICU later that night, I learned the child was doing fine. I can't say if the IV I started saved the child's life, but I do know it made a difference.

Reproduced with permission from Laustsen, G. (2005). Finely honed nursing skills. In S. Hudacek (Ed.), *Making a difference: Stories from the point of care* (Vol. 1, pp. 173–174). Indianapolis, IN: Sigma Theta Tau International.

EVIDENCE FOR PRACTICE

Guidelines from the Centers for Disease Control and Prevention (CDC, 2011) indicate peripheral IVs can remain in place 72 to 96 hours, as long as they are functioning properly and the patient is not showing signs of infection. An integrative review of the literature showed sutureless securement/stabilization

Continued

devices (e.g., StatLock) decrease complications associated with peripheral IV catheters and prolong their longevity and patency (Alekseyev et al., 2012). INS guidelines (2011) identify three types of products as acceptable for catheter stabilization:

- Manufactured catheter securement/stabilization devices (preferred).
- Sterile tapes.
- Surgical strips.

Table 5–1 Starting an IV Infusion

IV start kit (if available) *or:*
Tourniquet
Cleansing and antiseptic preparations
Dressings/transparent dressing (Opsite)
Small roll of sterile tape or sutureless catheter securement/stabilization device
Appropriate catheter for venipuncture: Determine size (gauge) by vein quality and size and anticipated infusion solutions; typical sizes for adults are 18-gauge or 20-gauge (higher number = smaller catheter size)
IV solution (if applicable)
IV tubing or pump and administration set (if applicable)
IV pole, rolling or ceiling-mounted
IV loop or short piece of extension tubing with 1–3 mL of sterile normal saline or heparin flush solution (per facility protocol) in syringe

ACTION STEPS	IMPORTANT NOTES
Verify the order and gather needed equipment and supplies. Wash your hands and explain the procedure to the patient.	Patient care: The size of the IV catheter may depend on expected therapeutics (e.g., blood administration or fluid rate). Having appropriate supplies at the bedside, such as extra needles or other equipment, allows you to be ready for multiple IV attempts. Many facilities use a prepackaged IV starter kit or have IV trays with needed supplies. The physician or advanced practice nurse will order the specific IV solution and flow rate. Make sure patients understand the purpose of their IV and how it will feel. Reinforce the need for their cooperation and not to move their extremity during the procedure.

Table 5–1 **Starting an IV Infusion—cont'd**

ACTION STEPS	IMPORTANT NOTES
Apply a tourniquet above the potential insertion site. Visualize and palpate for an appropriate vein.	The tourniquet should be tight enough to block venous return. Keep the tourniquet flat on the skin or on top of patient's gown. Put the arm in a dependent position. Warm towels may help distend veins if they are difficult to find. Having the patient open and close the fist may also help. Locating an IV site has many considerations. Nurses who excel at starting IV lines rely more on feeling for the vein than looking for one. They also apply knowledge of anatomy, physiology, and pathophysiology as they look for potential IV sites. Pick the nondominant arm if possible. Ask if the patient has had any lymph-node surgeries (e.g., mastectomy) on the arm; use the other arm if there is any concern about lymph system function in the arm. Try to find a site that allows the patient to have use of the hands. A site in the forearm (not on the medial aspect) is typically best. Avoid the wrist and antecubital areas. Try to find a vein that is straight and without junctions and that will accommodate the IV catheter size needed. Use a fingernail or pen top to make a small indentation at the preferred insertion site.
Release the tourniquet, prepare the equipment, reapply the tourniquet, don clean gloves, and clean the site (Fig. 5–1).	Leaving a tourniquet on for an extended time is painful for the patient and may alter laboratory results because of hemolysis. Place supplies within reach of one hand. If the patient is being readied for an IV fluid, prepare tubing and pump for immediate connection. Once equipment is ready,

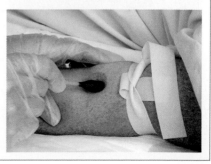

FIGURE 5–1: Cleaning IV insertion site.

Continued

Table 5–1 **Starting an IV Infusion—cont'd**

ACTION STEPS	IMPORTANT NOTES
	don clean gloves, and clean the insertion site per facility protocol, which may involve specific cleansing solutions (e.g., alcohol wipes or povidone-iodine). Wipe in a circular motion from the center outward. Once the site is clean, do not touch this area again.
Insert the IV catheter (Fig. 5–2).	Using your nondominant hand, pull the skin taut about 2 inches below the expected insertion site. Hold the IV needle hub in your dominant thumb and forefinger at a 10°–30° angle and bevel up. Insert the needle with a firm, smooth motion through the skin. When entering the vein, you may feel a "pop" or a change in resistance. Lower the angle, and advance the needle slightly into the vein. Look for blood return in the catheter chamber. Keep the needle steady, and advance the catheter with your nondominant hand into the vein to the hub. Release the tourniquet. Retract or remove the needle from the catheter while applying pressure on the skin above the end of the catheter. Attach IV tubing or an extension set. Test for flow through the tubing or, if using an extension set, flush with 3–5 mL of saline. Evaluate the insertion site for any signs of edema or infiltration. Dispose of the IV needle in the closest sharps container.

FIGURE 5–2: Inserting over-the-needle catheter.

Table 5-1 Starting an IV Infusion—cont'd

ACTION STEPS	IMPORTANT NOTES
Secure the IV catheter to the skin (Fig. 5–3).	Continue to hold the IV catheter hub and tubing securely. Clean with an alcohol swab any blood that may be near the insertion site. Secure the IV site as per protocol for your facility. At some agencies a clear, adhesive-backed covering (e.g., Opsite or Tegaderm) is placed on the skin over the IV hub and insertion site. The CDC recommends use of a catheter securement/stabilization device (e.g., StatLock). This device consists of an adhesive-backed anchor pad with hinged clamps that attach directly to the patient and swivel with patient movement. Loop the IV tubing up along the arm, and secure with nonallergenic tape.
Document the procedure, and monitor the IV site.	Label the site dressing with date and time per agency policy. Document in the patient record the date and time of IV placement. Include the size of the IV catheter and its location and how the patient tolerated the procedure. Monitor the IV site for signs of infection. If infusing fluids or medications, monitor for signs of infiltration.

FIGURE 5-3: Securing catheter and labeling site.

Inserting a Nasogastric Tube (NGT)

An NGT is a flexible plastic tube that passes through the nose, down the esophagus, and into the stomach. The NGT may facilitate:

- Infusing nutritional fluids
- Draining air or gastric secretions
- Irrigating the stomach
- Monitoring gastric bleeding

COACH CONSULT

Do you know why you hang the particular IV fluids that providers order for patients? Failure to master principles of IV fluid therapy can cause

Continued

149

COACH CONSULT —cont'd

complications, including death. Numerous factors influence the choice of IV fluids, including fluid, electrolyte, and acid-base imbalances. The following scenarios related to hypotonic and hypertonic IV fluids are adapted with permission from Laura Gasparis Vonfrolio, PhD, CEN, CCRN, RN:

- A 70-year-old woman is admitted to your unit with sepsis-dehydration. She has a history of heart failure (HF). Her blood pressure is 70/40. An order is given for 0.45% Saline at 75 mL an hour. Would you hang it?

No! The concentration of an IV solution is written on the front of the IV bag in mOSm/L. Check it before you hang it! Hypotonic solutions (less than 250 mOsm/L) such as 0.45% Saline (154 mOsm/L) shift fluid into the cells. Her blood pressure is already too low, which puts her at risk for acute renal failure. She needs all compartments hydrated with 0.9% Normal Saline (308 mOsm/L) to correct her dehydration and low blood pressure. Check her

Continued

Continued

EVIDENCE FOR PRACTICE

In a study using weight for the estimation of gastric tube insertion length in newborns, formulas were derived to predict tube insertion length in centimeters: orogastric = [3 × weight (kg) + 12] and nasogastric = [3 × weight (kg) + 13]. The formulas correctly predicted 60% of misplaced orogastric tubes and 100% of misplaced nasogastric tubes (Freeman et al., 2012).

NGT sizes range from 5 (small) to 18 (large) French. For adults, sizes 12 and above are typically used for stomach decompression or removal of gastric secretions. For long-term feeding, a smaller, specially designed NGT with a stylet (e.g., Dobhoff) is typically used. A critical aspect of NGT placement is verifying the tube is in the correct location. A misplaced NGT can result in serious patient harm, for example, if fluids are infused when an NGT has been inadvertently advanced into a lung. The increasing prevalence of bariatric surgery prompts nurses to consider additional safety implications of NGT placement. A 57-year-old woman who had undergone Roux-en-Y gastric bypass surgery 9 years earlier died because of perforation of the Roux limb of her gastric bypass. The perforation was caused by an NGT inserted for enteral nutrition, which resulted in fatal peritonitis detected on autopsy. Table 5–2 outlines the steps for inserting an NGT.

Inserting an Indwelling (Foley) Urinary Catheter

Many hospitalized patients require a temporary indwelling urinary catheter, often referred to by the brand name Foley. An indwelling urinary catheter:

- Allows drainage of urine if the patient cannot ambulate to the toilet or has urinary retention or incontinence.
- Facilitates bladder irrigation after surgery.
- Allows for monitoring of urinary output and the collection of urine samples for diagnostic purposes.
- May be used to instill fluid or dye for diagnostic purposes or warm fluid for removing blood clots or treating hypothermic patients.

Placement of a urinary catheter is an invasive procedure that can cause iatrogenic infections, so it is important for the nurse to perform the procedure with meticulous sterile technique, beginning with the foundational safety practice of hand hygiene. Another consideration is duration of catheterization, which is the most important risk factor for developing catheter-associated urinary tract infection (CAUTI). The size of the catheter chosen depends on patient size and reason for the catheter. Large catheters are common when irrigating the bladder after genitourinary surgery to allow passage of blood clots. Table 5–3 outlines the steps for inserting an indwelling (Foley) urinary catheter.

Administering a Blood Transfusion

Patients who have had significant blood loss from trauma, surgery, or internal bleeding may receive blood transfusions in addition to resuscitative crystalloid fluids. Blood products transfused may include whole blood, plasma, red blood cells (RBCs), or platelets. Although benchmarks now exist for blood transfusions,

COACH CONSULT —cont'd

blood pressure frequently and monitor her heart sounds for an S_3, which would indicate too much hydration given her history of HF.

- A 45-year-old man is admitted to your unit with a history of hypertension. Blood pressure on admission is 220/120. He has been on furosemide therapy and has severe intracellular dehydration. An order is given for Dextrose 5%–0.45% Saline (D5-1/2NS) at 50 mL an hour. Would you hang it?

No! The concentration of an IV solution is written on the front of the IV bag in mOSm/L. Check it before you hang it! Hypertonic solutions such as D5-1/2NS (406 mOsm/L) shift fluid out of cells. His blood pressure is already too high. He needs 0.45% Saline (154 mOsm/L) to shift fluids into his cells to correct his dehydration without increasing his blood pressure further.

Keep these principles of osmosis in mind when you hang IV fluids:

- Water moves across a semipermeable

Continued

protocols vary, and the nurse should always follow the individual institution's policy and procedures. For adults, blood should be infused through an IV line at least 20-gauge and preferably larger (18-gauge or 16-gauge). Frequent assessment of patients, during and after receiving blood products, is essential for monitoring for possible transfusion reactions. Table 5–4 outlines the steps for administering a blood transfusion.

Mixing Two Types of Insulin

Patients with diabetes may receive more than one type of insulin. Insulin types vary in their onset and duration of action and are generally classified as being short-acting, intermediate-acting, or long-acting. To minimize the need for multiple injections, nurses commonly seek to mix two types of insulin in the same syringe, but they must remember the following directives (see Evidence for Practice box and Table 5–5, "Mixing Insulin"):

- Lente insulins (Semilente, Lente, Ultralente) may be mixed with each other in any ratio.
- Lente and regular insulin generally should not be mixed with each other.
- Insulin glargine (Lantus) and insulin detemir (Levemir), both long-acting insulins, should not be mixed with any other insulin types.
- Neutral protamine Hagedorn (NPH) is the only long-acting insulin appropriate for mixing with short-acting insulins (i.e., regular, lispro, aspart, and glulisine insulins).
- To maintain the integrity and avoid cross-contamination of the multiuse vials of insulin, the nurse must follow the steps for

drawing each insulin type. While completing this procedure, the nurse should be aware of the institution's policy regarding a second nurse's verification of the insulin type and dose.

(Text continues on page 170)

EVIDENCE FOR PRACTICE

The journal *Diabetes Care* publishes research evidence and updates diabetes practice guidelines annually. Current best evidence for mixing insulin types reveals mixing lispro with glargine affects the pharmacodynamics of lispro. These changes potentially lead to difficulties in controlling meal-related glucose levels. Additionally, mixing aspart with detemir insulin markedly lowers the pharmacodynamics of the rapid-acting aspart and prolongs its duration compared with the separate injection of these analogs.

COACH CONSULT: READ MANUFACTURERS' DIRECTIONS—cont'd

actually cause damage to the balloon. It may also seem logical to inflate a 5-mL balloon with only 5 mL of sterile water from the prefilled 10-mL syringe and to assume the extra fluid is unnecessary or "just in case," such as improbable spillage. In fact, Bard's 5-mL balloon requires 9 to 10 mL of sterile water for sufficient inflation to prevent asymmetrical inflation of the balloon and to keep the catheter secure within the bladder and less likely to slip into the bladder neck.

Table 5–2 Inserting an NGT

NGT: Appropriate size (8–18 Fr) for patient (see NGT sizing below)
Nonallergenic tape (1 inch) or NGT anchoring device
Toomey syringe (20–60 mL)
Tincture of benzoin
Gloves (clean)
Water-soluble lubricant or topical anesthetic lubricant (Lidocaine)
pH paper
Safety pin
Cup of water and straw
Emesis basin
Penlight/flashlight
Stethoscope
Tissues
Tongue depressor
Wall or portable suction setup if ordered

Continued

Table 5–2 Inserting an NGT—cont'd

NGT SIZING
Adult: 14–18 Fr
To estimate NGT size for a pediatric patient, add 16 to the patient's age, and divide sum by 2. Choose a size closest to this value based on what is available. For example:
8 years old + 16/2 = 12 Fr
4 years old + 16/2 = 10 Fr
Infants: 5 or 8 Fr

ACTION STEPS	IMPORTANT NOTES
Verify the order, and gather needed equipment and supplies. Wash your hands, and explain the procedure to the patient.	Verify the reason the patient needs an NGT. The physician will order the correct type of NGT depending on purpose (feeding or decompression). The selection of NGT size is based on the size and age of the patient and the purpose for the NGT. NGT placement is often very uncomfortable for patients, although it should not be painful. Providing accurate information and answering patient questions can help decrease anxiety associated with this procedure. Especially inform patients not to pull the NGT out.
Assist the patient to a high Fowler's position (head of bed >45°). Ask the patient about any history of nasal surgery or trauma. Visually inspect each nasal vestibule for patency and an intact septum.	Upright positioning of the patient facilitates NGT placement and swallowing. Trauma or surgery of the nose may alter the ability of the NGT to pass through the nose. Establish a signal (e.g., patting own thigh with the hand) that the patient can use to signal you to pause the insertion.
Measure the NGT for length of insertion. Place the NGT end at the tip of the patient's nose, extend to the earlobe, and then extend to the xiphoid process. Mark this location with tape, or note the length mark on the NGT (Fig. 5–4).	The NGT needs to end in the patient's stomach, and this measurement will give you a close estimate of how far to insert the tube.

Table 5–2 Inserting an NGT—cont'd

ACTION STEPS	IMPORTANT NOTES

FIGURE 5–4: Measuring NGT for correct placement length.

ACTION STEPS	IMPORTANT NOTES
Give the patient a cup of water with a straw (if the patient may have fluids). Have facial tissues available for the patient. Keep an emesis basin nearby.	Having the patient sip water through a straw when asked will help advance the tube past the epiglottis. NGT placement often causes the patient's eyes to water, so use facial tissues to wipe away any tears. NGT placement may initiate gagging or vomiting.
Don clean gloves. Lubricate the tip of the NGT with water-soluble lubricant or anesthetic gel. Twist the tip of the NGT around your fingers to make a curl.	Lubrication with an anesthetic gel may provide some temporary numbing to the nasal mucosa. Some institutions may require a physician's order before using anesthetic gel. Twisting the NGT will help shape it to curve through the nasopharynx.
Have the patient raise his or her head up, and insert the NGT gently in an upward and backward direction. Do not use excessive force. Pause insertion when the tube reaches the pharynx.	Positioning the head of the patient helps straighten the nasal passage. Anticipate stimulating the gag reflex when the tube reaches the back of the oropharynx. Have the patient "pant like a puppy dog," which helps reduce gagging.

Continued

Table 5-2 Inserting an NGT—cont'd

ACTION STEPS	IMPORTANT NOTES
Have the patient lean his or her head forward to touch chin to chest. Advance the tube downward while the patient either swallows or sips water through a straw. Stop insertion if the patient needs a moment to breathe. Continue insertion until you reach the tape or mark on the NGT (Fig. 5–5).	Moving the head forward opens the esophagus, and swallowing helps to advance the tube. If the patient has excessive gagging or coughing, the tube may be curling in the back of the throat. If the patient experiences prolonged gagging, coughing, or dyspnea, remove the NGT immediately. Visualize the area with a penlight and tongue depressor. Twisting or rolling the tube between the fingers during insertion may help advance it. If gagging persists, remove the NGT. Once the NGT is in the stomach, gastric contents may start draining out. Connect the NGT to suction if ordered, or place the tip into an emesis basin.
Holding the NGT with one hand, aspirate stomach contents, and check the pH. Check centimeter markings on the NGT at the edge of the naris.	Stomach contents should be acidic (pH ≤4). Before taping, note the length measurement on the NGT at the edge of the naris. The NGT can migrate outward with time.

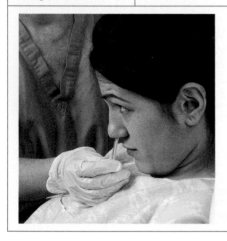

FIGURE 5–5: Lean head forward after NGT reaches the posterior pharynx.

Table 5-2 Inserting an NGT—cont'd

ACTION STEPS	IMPORTANT NOTES
Secure the NGT. Paint a small amount of tincture of benzoin on the nose. Split the bottom 1–2 inches of a piece of nonallergenic tape 3–4 inches long. Attach the unsplit end to the patient's nose. Wrap each split end around the NGT so that the tube is not against the skin of the naris. Secure the NGT to the patient's gown by attaching a safety pin through a piece of tape wrapped around the NGT. Use an NGT anchoring device if available (Fig. 5–6).	Benzoin helps keep the tape in place longer. Be careful not to get benzoin in the patient's eyes. Keep the NGT away from the edge of the nose to prevent tissue damage from rubbing. Attaching the NGT to the patient's gown minimizes the risk of snagging and pulling out the tube.

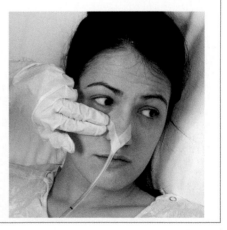

FIGURE 5-6: Securing NGT.

Continued

Table 5–2 Inserting an NGT—cont'd

ACTION STEPS	IMPORTANT NOTES
Connect the NGT to appropriate suction (if ordered). If a double-lumen NGT is used, place the vent cap into the vent tube. Order a chest x-ray to verify correct NGT placement before instilling anything in the tube. Document the procedure and the patient's response.	Physicians will order either continuous or intermittent suction (depending on tube type) for patients requiring removal of gastric secretions. A chest x-ray is the standard method for verifying correct placement of the NGT. You should receive confirmation from the physician or radiologist of correct tube placement before instilling anything through the NGT. Document in the patient record the size of the NGT, length of insertion, quantity and color of gastric contents, and how the patient tolerated the procedure.

Table 5–3 Inserting a Foley Catheter

Sterile urinary catheterization kit (kits may vary in their contents; the nurse should verify needed supplies for the procedure), which contains most of the following items:
Gloves
Drapes, one fenestrated
Lubricant
Antiseptic cleansing solution
Cotton balls
Forceps
Prefilled syringe with sterile water (inflates catheter balloon)
Catheter of correct size and type for procedure (extra catheters of same and smaller and larger sizes) (see important notes on appropriate size)
Sterile drainage tubing with collection bag
Securing device such as StatLock stabilization device or Velcro leg tube-holder Specimen container
The following items are not always included in the kit:
Extra pair or package of correct size sterile gloves
Blanket
Absorbent pad

ACTION STEPS	IMPORTANT NOTES
Verify the order, and gather needed equipment and supplies. Wash your hands, and explain the procedure to the patient.	Choose the equipment based on the patient's expected urethral size and the reason for the catheter. General size guidelines: 14–16 Fr for women

Table 5–3 Inserting a Foley Catheter—cont'd

ACTION STEPS	IMPORTANT NOTES
	12 Fr may be considered for young girls 16–18 Fr for men A physician may order a larger size for specific purposes (e.g., continuous bladder irrigation after surgery) or a smaller size for infants and small children.
Assess for allergies to antiseptic, tape, latex, and lubricant. Assess recent urinary symptoms or problems. Request assistance from another nurse or ancillary staff. Request others to leave the room, close the door, and draw the curtain. Warn the patient that you need to turn on a bright light and offer to cover his or her eyes with a dry washcloth.	Many patients are allergic to iodine-based cleaning solutions. Ask the patient about any past genital surgeries or previous experiences with catheters. Another nurse or medical assistant can be helpful with holding the patient's legs apart and aiding with equipment or the procedure itself. Patients generally desire privacy during this procedure.
Raise the bed to a comfortable working height. A right-handed nurse should do the procedure from the patient's right. Place the bedside stand with equipment at the end of the bed.	Typically, you insert the catheter while standing. The bed should be at a comfortable height. The head of the bed generally is flat or only slightly elevated.
Pull the bedding down to the foot of the bed. Position the patient with legs spread outward, knees bent, and feet together. Place a waterproof pad under the patient. Drape the patient with a bath blanket.	Appropriate positioning provides good visualization of the perineum area. Patients may need pillows or assistive personnel to support their legs. A warm blanket provides comfort and modesty for patients.
Wear clean gloves to wash and dry the perineal area. Remove gloves, and repeat hand hygiene.	Many patients may have soiled perineal areas because of incontinence or inability to perform adequate cleaning. Use warm, soapy water to clean the perineum, and dry well.
Open the catheterization kit on the bedside stand, maintaining a sterile field on the inner surface of the packaging.	The catheterization kit is often opened on a bedside stand but later transferred to the sterile pad on the bed. Maintain the sterility of the tray's bottom surface when opening the kit.

Continued

Table 5–3 Inserting a Foley Catheter—cont'd

ACTION STEPS	IMPORTANT NOTES
Place the underpad beneath the patient's buttocks. Don sterile gloves from the kit.	An underpad may or may not be in the tray. If not, use a clean, disposable underpad to protect the bedding under the patient.
Open the sterile package containing the catheter. Open the package of sterile antiseptic solution and pour it into the compartment with the sterile cotton balls. Open the lubricant packet. Set the specimen container aside. Attach the prefilled syringe to the catheter. Lubricate the catheter tip to a depth of 1–2 inches.	Check the catheter for integrity and kinks. Attach the prefilled syringe to the catheter and leave it in place. Squeeze the lubricant into the tray or, once open, place the packet over the end of the catheter.
Place the sterile drape on the bed between the patient's thighs, taking care not to touch any contaminated surface with sterile gloves. Place the fenestrated sterile drape over the perineum, exposing the patient's genitalia. Place the sterile tray and its contents on the sterile drape.	When placing the sterile drape, be careful not to touch the patient's legs or the bed with your sterile gloves. A fenestrated drape has a hole that opens over the genitalia. Move the tray to the sterile drape on the bed, being careful not to have it touch the patient's legs.
Female Catheterization	
With your nondominant hand, spread the labia to expose the urethral meatus, and hold this position throughout the procedure. With your dominant hand, use the forceps to pick up a cotton ball saturated with antiseptic solution. Clean the perineal area using a new cotton ball for each area. Wipe from front to back, clean the outer labial fold on each side, and then clean directly over the urethral meatus (Fig. 5–7).	Carefully position your nondominant hand, and spread the labia. This hand is now contaminated and needs to remain in place until the procedure is accomplished. After cleaning these areas, they become slippery, and it is difficult to respread the labia. Dispose of used cotton balls (after each wiping) away from the sterile field.
Pick up the lubricated catheter with your gloved dominant hand about 3–4 inches from the catheter tip. Ask the patient to bear down gently as if to void, and slowly insert the catheter through the urethral meatus. Advance the catheter 2–3 inches or until urine flows. When urine appears, advance the catheter 1–2 inches more. Do not force the catheter against resistance (Fig. 5–8).	Hold the catheter in your palm and the catheter tip with your thumb and index finger. Insert the catheter into the urinary meatus. If no urine appears, check if the catheter entered the vaginal opening below the meatus. If misplaced, leave the catheter in the vagina as a landmark indicating where *not* to insert.

Table 5–3 **Inserting a Foley Catheter—cont'd**

ACTION STEPS	IMPORTANT NOTES
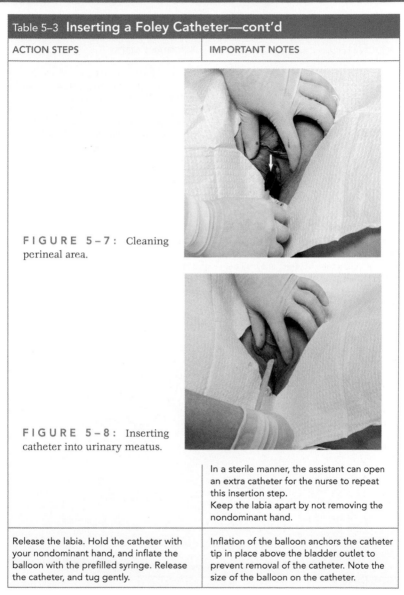 **FIGURE 5–7:** Cleaning perineal area. **FIGURE 5–8:** Inserting catheter into urinary meatus.	In a sterile manner, the assistant can open an extra catheter for the nurse to repeat this insertion step. Keep the labia apart by not removing the nondominant hand.
Release the labia. Hold the catheter with your nondominant hand, and inflate the balloon with the prefilled syringe. Release the catheter, and tug gently.	Inflation of the balloon anchors the catheter tip in place above the bladder outlet to prevent removal of the catheter. Note the size of the balloon on the catheter.

Continued

Table 5–3 Inserting a Foley Catheter—cont'd

ACTION STEPS	IMPORTANT NOTES
	A 5-mL balloon is most commonly used, and a prefilled syringe of 10 mL is included with the kit to fill the balloon to the appropriate size to keep the catheter in place. Use only the amount included. Do not overinflate or underinflate the balloon to prevent asymmetrical inflation. If you meet resistance during filling with the syringe, try advancing the catheter slightly. After filling the balloon, remove the syringe. Check that the catheter is secure in the bladder.
Secure the catheter tubing to the patient's inner thigh with a strip of nonallergenic tape or Velcro tube holders. Allow some slack in the tubing. Wash and dry the perineal area as needed to remove excess antiseptic solution (Fig. 5–9).	Velcro tube holders are more secure and less irritating than tape for securing catheter tubing. Excess antiseptic solution left at the site can cause itching and irritation.

FIGURE 5–9: Securing catheter to thigh.

Table 5-3 Inserting a Foley Catheter—cont'd

ACTION STEPS	IMPORTANT NOTES
Determine there is no urine leaking from the catheter or tubing connections. Document the procedure.	Assess the meatus area for signs of urine leakage or skin irritation, breakdown, or infection. Document in the patient record the size and type of catheter used, the balloon inflation volume (10 mL), the initial amount of urine that drained out, and how the patient tolerated the procedure.
Male Catheterization	
Follow all steps for Female Catheterization.	
Lift the patient's penis (upright in relation to the pelvis) with your nondominant hand, and retract the foreskin if the patient is uncircumcised. Use the forceps and three soaked cotton balls to clean the tip of the penis. Use a circular motion, and work outward from the meatus.	The nondominant hand is now considered contaminated.
Pick up the lubricated catheter with your gloved dominant hand about 3–4 inches from the catheter tip. Ask the patient to bear down gently as if to void, and slowly insert the catheter through the urethral meatus. Advance the catheter 6–8 inches or until urine flows. When urine appears, advance the catheter 1–2 inches more. Do not force the catheter against resistance (Fig. 5–10).	Some catheter trays have a syringe with lubricant that can be inserted directly into the meatus. Some resistance usually is felt at the area of the prostate, especially in older men. Twisting the catheter slightly during insertion may help it pass through the sphincters.
Release the penis, and hold the catheter with your nondominant hand. Inflate the balloon with the prefilled syringe. Release the catheter, and tug gently.	
Follow the final two steps under Female Catheterization.	In some men, securing the catheter with the penis directed toward the chest is more comfortable.

Continued

Table 5–3 Inserting a Foley Catheter—cont'd

ACTION STEPS	IMPORTANT NOTES

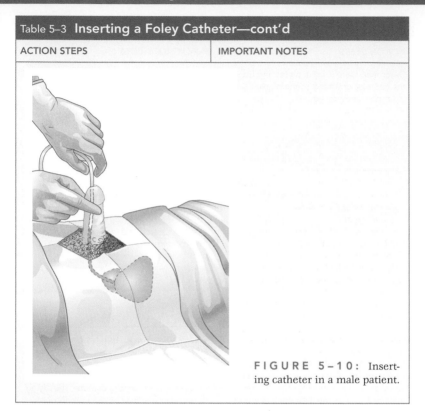

FIGURE 5–10: Inserting catheter in a male patient.

Table 5–4 Administering a Blood Transfusion

Blood product
Blood administration set (tubing with in-line filter and Y connector to saline)
250–500 mL normal (0.9%) saline solution
Gloves
Transfusion documentation forms
Optional: Additional 1,000 mL normal saline, tubing, and Y connector

ACTION STEPS	IMPORTANT NOTES
Verify the order, and gather needed equipment and supplies. Wash your hands,	Verify the correct time and date for infusion and type and amount of blood product

Table 5–4 Administering a Blood Transfusion—cont'd

ACTION STEPS	IMPORTANT NOTES
and explain the procedure to the patient. Verify the blood product and number of units or volume to be infused. Explain the procedure to the patient, and ask about any previous blood product transfusions and reactions.	ready for transfusion. Transfusion reactions are a potentially serious adverse event to blood product administration.
Verify patency of the current IV line. Administer any pretransfusion medications if ordered.	Flush the existing IV catheter with 3–5 mL of normal saline to verify patency. If the flow of the IV flush is slow or restricted, consider starting a new IV line. Physicians may order medications to minimize or prevent a transfusion reaction for patients with a history or potential for a transfusion reaction.
For whole blood, RBCs, or granulocytes, verify in the computer or with the blood bank: blood grouping, Rh type, number of units crossmatched, and number of units set up.	Administer the correct blood group and Rh type to avoid a transfusion reaction.
Except for emergency transfusions, verify that the patient has signed the informed consent. Check and verify the patient's hospital ID bracelet.	Administration of blood products requires informing the patient of risks and benefits of this procedure and having the patient sign a consent form acknowledging understanding of the procedure. This step may not be possible in emergency transfusions.
Obtain ordered blood product from the blood bank. Obtain and document baseline vital signs. Check the appearance of the blood product for the presence of clots, clumps, or abnormal cloudiness. Check the integrity of seals.	Administer blood products within 30 minutes of their leaving the blood bank refrigerator. Usually only one unit is released at a time. *Do not* place blood products from the blood bank in the refrigerator on the patient care unit. Return any blood products with an unusual appearance to the blood bank.

Continued

Table 5–4 Administering a Blood Transfusion—cont'd

ACTION STEPS	IMPORTANT NOTES
Before administration, two nurses trained in blood administration procedures compare (1) the blood product from the blood bank with the product requested in the physician's order; (2) blood type and Rh type recorded for the patient with the container bag and label, verifying that they are identical or compatible; (3) the blood product number on the blood bag with the product number on the blood bag tag; and (4) the expiration date and time on the blood container label with the current date and time (Fig. 5–11).	All records must correspond exactly. All identification attached to the blood container bag must remain attached until completion of the transfusion.
In the presence of the recipient and immediately before the transfusion, two nurses identify the patient using at least two forms of identification: (1) compare and verify the patient's name and medical record number on the blood unit with the recipient's identification bracelet and the information recorded in the patient record; (2) ask the patient to state his or her name.	Wrong patient, wrong blood product, and other identification errors are the most common causes of adverse transfusion events. Checking for the correct patient is a *critical* step in the transfusion process. For any discrepancy, notify the blood bank, and return the blood product until the problem is resolved.

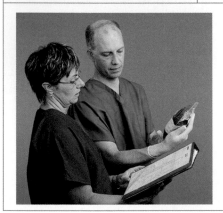

FIGURE 5–11: Verifying blood product with two RNs.

Table 5–4 Administering a Blood Transfusion—cont'd

ACTION STEPS	IMPORTANT NOTES
Prime the blood tubing administration set with the blood product or normal saline (Fig. 5–12).	Consider adding a three-way stopcock onto the end of the blood administration set, and have a bag of normal saline and IV tubing available for emergency use or attached to the stopcock. Use a blood warmer if needed. *Do not* microwave blood products.
For adults, adjust the rate of flow to 2–5 mL/min for the first 5 minutes for platelet or plasma infusions or 2 mL/min for the first 15 minutes for whole blood, RBCs, or granulocytes. Observe the patient closely for the first 15 minutes.	An infusion pump may facilitate administration of blood products. Adverse reactions usually occur during infusion of the initial 50 mL. Careful monitoring for a reaction can decrease patient complications or death. Typical reaction symptoms include flushing, dyspnea, itching, hives, or a rash.

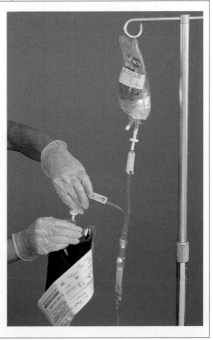

FIGURE 5–12: Priming blood tubing.

Continued

Table 5–4 Administering a Blood Transfusion—cont'd

ACTION STEPS	IMPORTANT NOTES
After 15 minutes, obtain and record a full set of vital signs. If vital signs are within the normal range and the patient has no signs and symptoms of an adverse reaction, change the infusion rate to the physician-prescribed time period. Continue monitoring the patient for adverse reactions up to 1 hour after transfusion. If you suspect a transfusion reaction, immediately stop the transfusion. Maintain patency of the IV line by infusing normal saline, and notify the physician.	Adverse transfusion reactions can occur anytime during or after the transfusion. If a transfusion reaction occurs, do not discard the blood products. Save them for analysis.
After blood product transfusion, flush the blood administration set with normal saline until the tubing is clear. Obtain and document vital signs. Disconnect and discard the empty blood product bag into a biohazard receptacle. Document the transfusion in the patient record and return the transfusion documentation forms to the patient's chart and blood bank as required by facility policy.	If required to administer additional transfusions, check the institution's policy about reusing blood tubing sets. Documentation should include the time and date of transfusion, the type and amount of blood product transfused, transfusion vital signs, and the patient's response to the transfusion. Patients should be monitored after the transfusion for the potential of fluid overload.

Table 5–5 Mixing Insulin

Insulin syringe and needle: Syringe must be appropriate size for total amount of insulin. Vials of two insulin types.

ACTION STEPS	IMPORTANT NOTES
Verify the order, and gather needed equipment and supplies. Wash your hands.	Insulin comes in many forms, and patients with diabetes are on a wide range of dosages. Make sure insulin types and amount are correct. Insulin syringes usually have the needle attached and come in various sizes (30, 50, and 100 units). Choose a syringe size that will contain the entire amount of both insulin doses and that you can read accurately. The needle length also

Table 5–5 Mixing Insulin—cont'd

ACTION STEPS	IMPORTANT NOTES
	varies; you should select a needle that reaches adequately into the subcutaneous space. Needles come in lengths of ³⁄₁₆ inch, ⁵⁄₁₆ inch, and ½ inch.
For new vials, remove the plastic cap. For insulin suspensions (NPH), roll the vial between your hands to mix well. There is no need to roll or mix "clear" insulins. Set the insulin vials on a flat counter, and clean the tops of the vials with alcohol swabs.	Mix insulin in suspension before withdrawing it from the vial. NPH is the only insulin currently produced in suspension. Do not shake the vial.
Inject air into the nonregular insulin equal to the amount of units you will remove. Do not let the needle touch the vial contents. Touch the plunger knob only to avoid contamination of the syringe barrel. Withdraw the syringe from the nonregular insulin vial, and inject air into the regular insulin equal to the amount of units you will remove. Do not remove the needle (Fig. 5–13).	The goal in this technique is to prevent long-acting insulin from contaminating insulin in the short-acting vial. In the past, nurses used such phrases as "clear to cloudy" to remember the order for drawing up two types of insulin. Because newer long-acting insulins are not all cloudy, remember the phrase: "short to long" instead.
Invert the regular insulin vial, and remove the ordered amount of regular insulin. Have a second nurse verify the correct insulin type and dose. Remove the needle from the regular insulin vial, insert it into the nonregular insulin vial, invert, and withdraw the ordered amount of nonregular insulin into the syringe. Again, have a second nurse verify the correct insulin type and dose (see Fig. 5–13).	Because of the significant action of insulin and potential for error in drawing up the drug, institutions generally require two nurses to check insulin doses before injecting them into the patient. The needle must stay in the bottle until the second nurse has verified the type *and* amount of insulin. Repeat this step after you draw up the second type of insulin.
Carefully recap the needle. Return the insulin vials to their appropriate storage location. Explain what you are doing, and administer the mixed insulin to the patient. Document the drug administration (see Fig. 5–13).	Unless you mix the insulins at the bedside, recap the needle. Using a built-in protector or recapping device or approved method protects you and others from an accidental needle-stick. Many facilities and patients keep insulin refrigerated, although it keeps at room temperature for up to 1 month after opening. Injection of room-temperature insulin is less irritating to the patient.

Continued

169

Table 5–5 Mixing Insulin—cont'd

ACTION STEPS	IMPORTANT NOTES

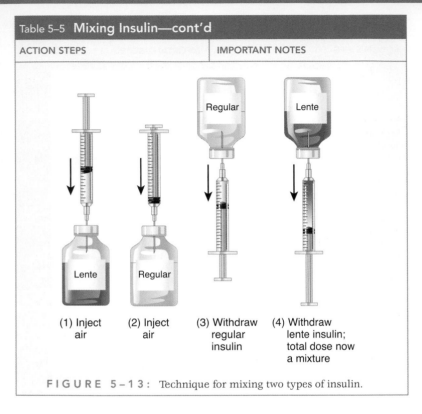

(1) Inject air   (2) Inject air   (3) Withdraw regular insulin   (4) Withdraw lente insulin; total dose now a mixture

FIGURE 5–13: Technique for mixing two types of insulin.

Performing Tracheostomy Care

A tracheostomy is a surgical opening of the trachea to provide and secure an open airway. A trained health-care professional inserts a tube in the anterior portion of the neck through a stoma in the cricoid cartilage, directly into the trachea. Patients may have a tracheostomy for a number of reasons:

- To provide an emergency airway when facial trauma or illness occludes the upper airway.
- To provide a long-term or permanent airway in an intubated patient who does not have full respiratory ability.

In contrast to an endotracheal tube, a tracheostomy may allow the patient to talk and eat. The tracheostomy, or "trach," tube is typically a curved plastic device (inner cannula) that inserts into a hard plastic outer cannula with a flat plastic collar or flange. The tube is available in many sizes and may be cuffed or uncuffed. An obturator fits into the inner cannula during insertion. Trach tape, a tie, or a padded strap around the neck secures the trach tube. Patients with a tracheostomy need frequent care of the tube because the insertion site gives potential access for infection of the respiratory system. Tracheal tissue necrosis is also a potential problem associated with cuffed trach tubes. See Table 5–6 for steps used in performing tracheostomy care.

EVIDENCE FOR PRACTICE

About a decade ago, the Nursing Performance Improvement and Nursing Research departments at Walter Reed Army Medical Center entered into a research collaboration to facilitate evidence-based practice better. Their pilot project on tracheostomy care included grading more than 30 articles using Agency for Healthcare Research and Quality levels of evidence and resulted in a tracheostomy care and suctioning algorithm, which continues to represent the state of the science. The success of this initiative prompted similar efforts for pressure ulcer prevention, deep vein thrombosis prophylaxis, and enteral feeding. The two departments also modeled an effective way for nurses to collaborate across an institution to achieve quality outcomes and improve patient safety (St. Clair, 2005).

Table 5–6 Performing Tracheostomy Care

Towel
Tracheostomy suction supplies
Hydrogen peroxide
Normal saline (NS)
Scissors
Two sterile gloves
Face shield, if indicated
Sterile tracheostomy care kit, if available, *or:*
Three sterile 4 × 4 gauze pads
Sterile cotton-tipped applicators
Sterile tracheostomy dressing
Sterile basin

Continued

Table 5–6 Performing Tracheostomy Care—cont'd

Small sterile brush (or disposable cannula)
Tracheostomy ties (e.g., twill tape, manufactured tracheostomy ties, Velcro tracheostomy strap)

ACTION STEPS	IMPORTANT NOTES
Verify the order, and gather needed equipment and supplies. Wash your hands, and explain the procedure to the patient. Perform care as needed if the tube is unstable or has become soiled with excess secretions. Obtain a tracheostomy care kit and any additional supplies. Assess the patient's respiratory status. Suction the tracheostomy, and remove the old dressing. Keep an oxygen source available during the procedure.	Patients with tracheostomy tubes are at increased risk for airway complications because normal protective mechanisms have been bypassed. Maintain aseptic technique during tracheostomy care. Removing any secretions will decrease potential aspiration or outer cannula blockage. Stabilize the tracheostomy tube during care to prevent dislodgment, injury, or discomfort. Before, during, or after care, patients may experience oxygen desaturation. Keep appropriate oxygen delivery devices available, and consider using "blow-by" oxygen during the tracheostomy procedure.
Open two packages of cotton-tipped swabs. Add NS to one package and hydrogen peroxide to the other. Keep hydrogen peroxide and saline solutions open for future use. Open a sterile tracheostomy package. Unwrap a sterile basin, and pour a small amount of hydrogen peroxide into it. Open a small sterile brush package, and place it into the sterile basin. Don sterile gloves, and maintain sterility of your dominant hand.	Hydrogen peroxide solution helps loosen secretions. NS helps remove any potentially irritating hydrogen peroxide. Maintain sterility of solution bottles by not allowing the top of the bottle to touch any supplies or surfaces. Tracheostomy kits may contain sterile gloves; however, they may not be your size. Always have available at least one extra set of sterile gloves.
To replace a *disposable inner cannula,* do as follows. Remove new cannula from packaging (Fig. 5–14). Touching only the outer aspect of the tracheostomy tube, unlock and remove the old inner cannula, and replace it with the new one. Lock the new cannula into position.	Either after a certain period or with certain types of cannulas, replace the inner cannula rather than clean it. Follow guidelines of the physician, institution, or manufacturer for when to replace the inner cannula.

Table 5–6 Performing Tracheostomy Care—cont'd

ACTION STEPS	IMPORTANT NOTES

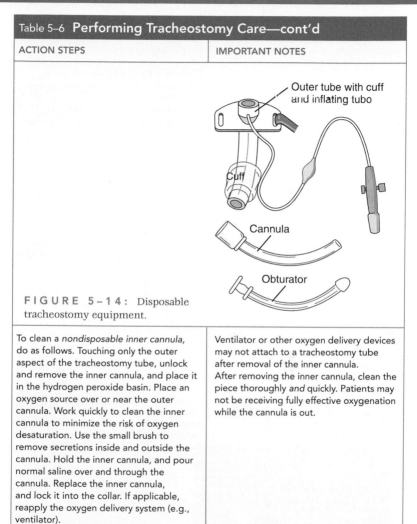

Outer tube with cuff and inflating tubo

Cuff

Cannula

Obturator

FIGURE 5 – 14: Disposable tracheostomy equipment.

ACTION STEPS	IMPORTANT NOTES
To clean a *nondisposable inner cannula,* do as follows. Touching only the outer aspect of the tracheostomy tube, unlock and remove the inner cannula, and place it in the hydrogen peroxide basin. Place an oxygen source over or near the outer cannula. Work quickly to clean the inner cannula to minimize the risk of oxygen desaturation. Use the small brush to remove secretions inside and outside the cannula. Hold the inner cannula, and pour normal saline over and through the cannula. Replace the inner cannula, and lock it into the collar. If applicable, reapply the oxygen delivery system (e.g., ventilator).	Ventilator or other oxygen delivery devices may not attach to a tracheostomy tube after removal of the inner cannula. After removing the inner cannula, clean the piece thoroughly *and* quickly. Patients may not be receiving fully effective oxygenation while the cannula is out.

Continued

Table 5–6 Performing Tracheostomy Care—cont'd

ACTION STEPS	IMPORTANT NOTES
Clean the stoma, skin, and outer surfaces of the tracheostomy tube and faceplate. Work outward from the stoma, using swabs and gauze soaked in hydrogen peroxide. Rinse all areas with swabs and gauze soaked in NS. Dry the skin and outer tracheostomy surfaces by patting them lightly with a 4 × 4 gauze pad.	Clean from the stoma area outward to minimize introducing infectious agents into the stoma opening. After cleaning, dry all wet surfaces to minimize growth of bacteria and to protect the skin from excoriation.
Replace ties and dressing. If available, have an assistant hold the tracheostomy tube, and cut the old ties. If assistance is not available, attach new ties before removing the old ones. Cut tracheostomy or twill tape on a diagonal with enough length to encircle the patient's neck two times: about 2–2½ feet for an adult. Insert the cut end into one side of the faceplate, and adjust until the ends are about even. Slide the tie around behind the patient's neck, and thread the cut end through the other eyelet on the faceplate. Secure the ends of the tie with a double square knot, allowing enough slack between the tie and the neck for one finger. Cut any excess tie (Fig. 5–15). Replace the old tracheostomy dressing with a new dressing under the faceplate.	Accidental extubation is a risk during care and especially while replacing ties. A new tracheostomy tube of the same size and obturator should be available at the patient's bedside in case of emergency replacement. Temporarily insert a size 6 endotracheal tube in the stoma if a replacement tube is not readily available. Making diagonal cuts on the end of the tracheostomy tie makes it easier to insert the tie through the eyelet. The slack allows space for the new tracheostomy dressing. The dressing helps absorb secretions or drainage and minimizes pressure on the clavicle heads. Always use a tracheostomy-specific dressing. *Do not* take regular 4 × 4 gauze and cut a groove in it to slip around the tube. Small loose fibers from the cut edges may enter the patient's airway.

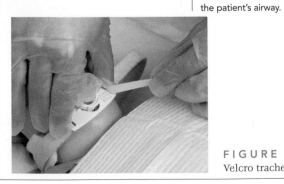

FIGURE 5–15: Securing Velcro tracheostomy tie.

Table 5–6 Performing Tracheostomy Care—cont'd

ACTION STEPS	IMPORTANT NOTES
Reassess the patient's respiratory status, and compare findings with the patient's preprocedure status. Assess other aspects of the patient's response, and document the procedure.	Monitor the patient's tolerance of the procedure and respiratory status (oxygen saturation via pulse oximetry, lung sounds, and respiratory rate and effort). Suction as needed after completing the procedure.

Taking Orthostatic Vital Signs

Patients may become hypovolemic (volume-depleted) because of blood or plasma loss, dehydration, or dilation of peripheral blood vessels (e.g., in neurogenic shock). These patients are not able to compensate and maintain a stable heart rate (HR) and blood pressure (BP) when changing positions from supine to either sitting or standing. Taking orthostatic vital signs, sometimes called "posturals" or the tilt test, helps to identify patients who may be hypovolemic. However, orthostatic vital signs alone lack the sensitivity to detect reliably volume losses less than 1,000 mL. Symptoms such as dizziness and syncope, in combination with orthostatic vital signs, are more sensitive indicators of volume loss than vital sign changes alone. In particular, changes in BP and pulse need to be considered in relation to the patient's past and current medical history, medication use, time of day, recent oral intake, and age.

The procedure for taking orthostatic vital signs has moderate support from an integrative review of the literature (Naccarato et al., 2012). It is recommended that a patient should be supine 5 to 10 minutes before beginning the series of vital signs. Position change from supine to standing has better diagnostic accuracy in volume-depleted adults compared with position change from supine to sitting and then to standing. Blood pressure measurements should be taken at 1 minute and 3 minutes after standing.

Standards vary regarding the vital sign changes needed to consider a patient orthostatic or to have a positive tilt test. The literature provides moderate support for clinicians who use the 20-10-20 guideline to describe a positive test: a 20-point change in systolic BP, a 10-point change in diastolic BP, and a 20-point change in pulse rate (Naccarato et al., 2012). See Table 5–7 for steps in taking orthostatic vital signs.

Table 5–7 Taking Orthostatic Vital Signs

Stethoscope
Blood pressure cuff (appropriate size for patient's arm)
Sphygmomanometer or electronic BP device
Watch with second hand

ACTION STEPS	IMPORTANT NOTES
Verify the order, and gather needed equipment and supplies. Wash your hands, and explain the procedure to the patient. Verify the BP cuff size is correct for the patient's arm diameter.	To avoid possible equipment errors, it is best to use the same equipment each time you take vital signs. BP cuffs that are the wrong size may give either falsely high or falsely low readings. Explain the process to the patient. It is especially important that patients tell you if they feel dizzy, lightheaded, faint, or nauseated when changing positions. Patients may faint, fall, and hurt themselves while you obtain these vital signs.
Put the patient in a supine position for at least 10 minutes. If this position compromises respiratory function, raise the head of the bed slightly.	Keeping the patient supine for 10 minutes allows the BP to equilibrate to this position after the patient has been moved from a different position.
Place the BP cuff on the patient's arm, and either start the electronic device or take a manual BP. Take the patient's radial pulse rate, or read it from the electronic device.	Use the same arm and pulse site each time you take orthostatic vital signs. Electronic devices produce consistent results and avoid possible bias or poor technique of the person taking the vital signs.
Leave the BP cuff on, and assist the patient to the new position (sitting, if warranted for safety or other reasons, or standing). Repeat vital signs at 1 minute and at 3 minutes. Ask the patient to report any dizziness, and monitor for clinical signs of near-syncope (e.g., pale skin, lack of response to questions). *Note:* If checking all three positions, assist the patient to a standing position, and repeat the vital signs at 1 minute and at 3 minutes. Continue to monitor for clinical signs of near-syncope, and return the patient to bed if any risk of fainting.	Moving the patient from supine to standing and taking two readings is more common than taking a second reading while the patient is sitting and a third while standing. Some patients may be unable to stand, requiring the second reading in a sitting position. Monitor the patient carefully while getting the vital signs. A patient may not warn of feeling faint before collapsing. Be especially careful with patients who are heavy or unsteady on their feet. For electronic medical records that have space for all three positions, take the readings supine, standing, and sitting.

Table 5–7 Taking Orthostatic Vital Signs—cont'd

ACTION STEPS	IMPORTANT NOTES
Document findings in the chart. Call the provider immediately if results are significant or if the patient experienced severe dizziness. Documentation may include line figures to represent the various positions. Document any subjective comments the patient makes.	Use the 20-10-20 guideline to describe a positive test: a 20-point change in systolic BP, a 10-point change in diastolic BP, and a 20-point change in pulse rate. Sample documentation with positive orthostatic vital signs: BP = 140/80; HR = 64 (supine) BP = 128/88; HR = 76 (sitting) BP = 112/92; HR = 90 (standing) "I feel dizzy."

Performing an Electrocardiogram (ECG)

According to the CDC, the procedure for performing an ECG has been unchanged for 2 decades. An ECG is a procedure that produces a printout (sometimes called a 12-lead) of the electrical activity of the heart. Recording an ECG involves placing multiple electrodes on each of a patient's four limbs and in specific locations on the chest wall (precordium). Each combination of electrodes used in standard electrocardiography is called a lead. A 12-lead ECG creates a view of the heart's electrical impulses from 12 different combinations of leads and prints these waveforms on graph paper moving at a set rate through the ECG machine. An ECG recording represents a view of the heart's electrical activity for only a few seconds. Standard ECGs are also limited in that they do not show the right and posterior aspects of the heart very well. A 15-lead or 18-lead ECG is sometimes requested by the provider to look for possible involvement of the right ventricular and posterior aspects of the heart. A standardized ECG machine may be used for 15-lead or 18-lead ECGs with repositioning of the six chest (V) leads by the nurse.

Although many facilities have ECG technicians who routinely perform ECGs, nurses should familiarize themselves with both performing and reading ECGs. Nurses should also advocate for safe, cost-effective, and evidence-based practice related to ECGs, including:

- Adherence to clinical guidelines, for example, in the case of chest pain, ECG recording, and patient assessment within 10 minutes of arrival in an emergency department.

- Consistent skin preparation and the use of electrode impedance meters to minimize interference that changes ECG morphology.
- The use of ECG in the diagnosis and management of heart failure.

A physician or advanced practice nurse is responsible for the official ECG interpretation. Nurses, especially in critical care areas, should be able to read and identify ECGs that indicate serious problems such as myocardial infarction (MI). Nurses working in critical care areas typically are required to attend classes in basic and advanced ECG interpretation. Table 5–8 outlines the steps for performing an ECG.

Table 5–8 Performing an ECG

ECG machine
Self-adhesive, disposable monitor lead electrodes
Gauze pads
Extra blanket
Electric razor (optional)

ACTION STEPS	IMPORTANT NOTES
Verify the order, and gather needed equipment and supplies. Wash your hands, and explain the procedure to the patient.	Many patients are unfamiliar with this procedure. The presence of so many wires can be concerning or frightening. Reassure the patient that no electricity will be in the wires, which detect or "read" the heart's electrical activity.
Position the patient supine, if possible, with arms at the sides and legs uncrossed. If the supine position causes respiratory difficulties, put the patient in a Fowler's or upright position. Close the room door or pull the bed curtain to provide privacy. Pull the patient's gown down to the waist. Female patients may need to remove their bra.	Assist the patient into a relaxed position.
Place the 10 electrodes on the patient's arms, legs, and chest as indicated in Figure 5–16. Choose flat, fleshy areas; avoid bony or muscular areas. If the skin is sweaty or oily, wiping with gauze pads will help electrodes stick better. Clip areas of	Placement of the electrodes and attachment of the leads to the correct electrode are *critical* to obtaining an accurate ECG. Lead wires have letters indicating the location: RA means right arm, LL means left leg. Each of the six chest

Table 5–8 Performing an ECG—cont'd

ACTION STEPS	IMPORTANT NOTES

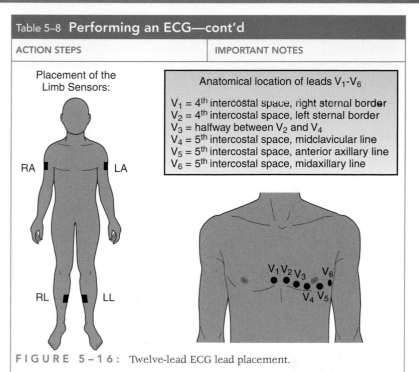

Placement of the Limb Sensors:

RA   LA

RL   LL

Anatomical location of leads V_1-V_6

V_1 = 4th intercostal space, right sternal border
V_2 = 4th intercostal space, left sternal border
V_3 = halfway between V_2 and V_4
V_4 = 5th intercostal space, midclavicular line
V_5 = 5th intercostal space, anterior axillary line
V_6 = 5th intercostal space, midaxillary line

V_1 V_2 V_3 V_6
        V_4 V_5

FIGURE 5–16: Twelve-lead ECG lead placement.

thick hair with an electric razor to allow each electrode to adhere adequately. Attach the 10 leads to the correct electrodes.	leads (V1–V6) has a specific anatomic location for correct placement. Do not use a razor blade to shave the hair because of the potential for minor skin lacerations. Place electrodes under the breast in women. Point leg leads superiorly.
After attaching lead wires to the electrodes, assess the patient. If the patient is cold and shivering, gently place a blanket for warmth. Turn on the ECG machine, and enter the appropriate patient data. Ask the patient to relax, to breathe slowly, and not to talk. Press the AUTO button; the ECG machine will automatically read and produce the 12-lead ECG tracing. Review the tracing for quality.	Muscular contractions from shivering or trembling will interfere with producing a good ECG recording. Most ECG machines indicate appropriate lead connection but not correct location. Poor waveforms may be due to patient movement, deep breathing, or talking or to poor lead placement.

Continued

Table 5–8 **Performing an ECG—cont'd**	
ACTION STEPS	IMPORTANT NOTES
If the tracing appears adequate, transmit or save the ECG data as required by protocol, remove the electrodes from the patient, and replace the patient's gown. Document in the patient record the ECG procedure and the patient's response.	Many patients will ask the person doing the ECG, "Is everything OK?" Current protocols generally require interpretation by a cardiologist, other physician, or qualified advanced practice nurse. Inform patients that their provider or cardiologist will review, interpret, and discuss the results of the ECG with them.

Managing Basic Bedside Monitoring

Whether used on an intermittent or continuous basis, a portable bedside monitor (Fig. 5–17) facilitates obtaining and recording basic patient parameters, such as BP, HR, temperature, respiratory rate, oxygen saturation, and cardiac rhythm. Nurses often print data directly from the machine for documentation purposes.

Continuous monitoring is a key activity in the surveillance process, but monitoring alone is insufficient for the provision of safe, high-quality bedside care. The term surveillance refers to purposeful and ongoing acquisition, interpretation, and synthesis of patient data for clinical decision making. Regardless of the reasons for using a bedside monitor, nurses must verify the following:

- Accuracy of readings: Calibrate devices as needed, and verify movement-based data.
- Appropriateness of alarms: Set appropriate minimum and maximum levels for each patient; turn alarms on for all devices in use.

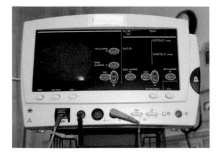

FIGURE 5–17: Patient bedside monitor.

- Agreement with actual patient status: Acknowledge limitations of bedside monitors, verify placement of devices, and obtain subjective data.
- Documentation of verified data: Enter applicable data in the patient's medical record.

Table 5–9 outlines the basics of bedside monitoring.

Table 5–9 Basic Bedside Monitoring

BLOOD PRESSURE	• Bedside patient monitors are usually capable of obtaining noninvasive blood pressure (NIBP) readings. As with a manual BP, select an appropriate-sized cuff for accurate BP determination. Patient movement may affect readings. Check and reposition the cuff occasionally for patient comfort, skin assessment, and reading accuracy. • For continuous monitoring, set the monitor to record NIBPs at appropriate intervals (e.g., every 5, 10, 15, or 60 minutes), subject to change depending on findings for a given patient. Too frequent inflation may be uncomfortable for the patient and may falsely elevate the BP. • Set the monitor to alarm when the NIBP is outside the high or low limits for both the systolic and the diastolic BP readings, according to the patient's past readings and condition.
HEART RATE	• Bedside monitors record heart rate (HR) by measuring the pulse rate either from the pulse oximeter or from the cardiac rhythm leads. • For HRs measured by pulse oximeter, inaccuracies may occur with poor circulation because of cold extremities or compromised vasculature or with poor waveforms on the monitor. • For HRs obtained from the cardiac monitor, the leads pick up the electrical signals of the heart and convert those signals into a rhythm tracing. From the tracings, the monitor reads the number of individual beats per minute to display the HR. The display of the HR on a monitor changes frequently. Determine an average of these changing numbers when recording the HR. • For either method, verify that (1) alarms are set and on for minimum and maximum HR according to the patient's condition (values may need adjustment with changes in patient status or care, such as addition of medications that affect HR) and (2) displayed values are accurate. Perform a manual pulse rate according to agency protocol or at least once per shift.

Continued

Table 5–9 Basic Bedside Monitoring—cont'd

TEMPERATURE	• Some bedside monitors have a built-in temperature recording parameter. A dedicated wire from the monitor connects to a skin temperature recording device, a specialized urinary catheter, or a rectal probe. • Continuous temperature monitoring may be important for monitoring neurologically unstable, hyperthermic, or hypothermic patients. • Temperature probes require accurate placement to achieve reliable results.
RESPIRATORY RATE	When patients have cardiac rhythm leads in place, their respiratory rate displays according to changes in two leads during the rise and fall of the chest wall. Many patients do not have enough change in elevation of their chest wall during respirations for detection by the leads, so the displayed respiratory rate is often inaccurate. Respiratory rates obtained from bedside monitors require in-person observation to confirm their accuracy.
OXYGEN SATURATION VIA PULSE OXIMETRY	• A pulse oximeter has a probe, typically placed on a finger, to read the percent of oxygenation in the blood. The infrared light in the probe evaluates the amount of blood that is saturated (typically with oxygen) and records the pulse rate. • Pulse oximeter probes depend on correct placement in an appropriate location. For adults, the thumb or index finger is usually suitable. In young children, the top of the foot or big toe is often a good location. Special single-use tape-on probes facilitate continuous monitoring via pulse oximetry in pediatric patients. • The display on the monitor includes an oxygen saturation percentage, pulse rate, and a visual waveform. The waveform gives an indication of the strength of the pulse and helps you evaluate the reliability of the displayed readings. If the waveform is not strong or the pulse rate is not accurate, you should be suspicious of the oxygen saturation reading. • Like the HR display, the pulse oximetry display will change frequently over time. Set the alarm to sound when the oxygen saturation falls below a predetermined level.
CARDIAC RHYTHM	• Bedside monitors are often capable of displaying a single-lead ECG. Most monitors rely on three or five wires (leads) for placement at specific locations on the patient to record the electrical signals from the heart. The nurse or ECG technician attaches leads to self-adhesive monitor patches

Table 5–9 Basic Bedside Monitoring—cont'd

	that adhere to a patient's chest. Depending on the location of the lead wires and the setting of the monitor, the display may be able to show more than one ECG view. In one common view, called lead II, the technician or nurse places leads on the upper right and upper left chest and on the lower left abdomen, hip, or thigh. This arrangement of leads produces the common cardiac tracing of an upright QRS (if the patient has a normal sinus rhythm).

- Lead wires typically follow a color-coded protocol, with the upper right wire white, the upper left wire black, and the lower abdomen wire either green or red. Some nurses learn the memory device "White is right and smoke over fire" to remember proper placement of the different lead wires. The lead wires on some monitors are replaceable, however, which can result in incorrect placement when replaced. A better method is to note the plug holding the lead wires, which always has RA (right arm), LA (left arm), and LL (left lower) on it so you can accurately place the leads in the correct location regardless of the color of the lead wire.
- In addition to setting alarms for minimum and maximum HR, many bedside monitors can sound an alarm when certain ECG tracings occur, such as ventricular tachycardia, ventricular fibrillation, or multiple ectopic beats.

Chapter Summary

This chapter focused on nine critical skills of patient care and provided essential details to help you master them. Being articulate about the action steps and associated elements will help you accelerate your own path to nursing competency, recognition, and promotion. In Chapter 6, we support the critical thinking and clinical judgment needed to deliver safe, outcome-driven patient care through an in-depth examination of shift planning.

6 Shift Planning: Conquering Shift Organization and Prioritization

CHAPTER 6

Shift Planning: Conquering Shift Organization and Prioritization

This chapter accelerates your mastery of "shifting." Although your shifts will not become automatic, a well-organized shift promotes optimal patient outcomes by means of planning and confident prioritization. A carefully crafted shift also acknowledges and accommodates the flexibility needed to respond to rapidly changing patient and unit conditions. To reach the destination of desired patient and organizational outcomes, we draw on all standards of the nursing process and several tested methods, such as comprehensive shift organizers and sample clinical scenarios.

Planning your shift is one of the most important things you can do to provide safe, quality patient care. This standard of the nursing process taps into multiple ways of thinking, described in Chapter 1, to help you cope with the reality that every shift and every patient assignment vary. As part of your shift planning and organization, we review how to give an organized end-of-shift report and how to make the beginning and end of your shift a smooth hand-off for you and others on the next shift. Remember, we are all on one team, even when we work different shifts.

COACH CONSULT

To achieve desired outcomes, we encourage you to go the extra mile: Before each shift, think about, visualize, and feel the joy of making a difference in the lives of your patients. Your colleagues may not know your secret, but they will say you bring "something extra" to your nursing care.

Equally important, being able to modify the plan appropriately is the hallmark of a professional in any field. Evaluation, another standard of the nursing process, derives from clinical reasoning and judgment about your nursing care plan and available data. Much like anticipating potholes on the road, anticipating and recognizing shift anomalies—and knowing how to rebound from them—can assist you in maintaining or adapting your plan of care. We include a table of common shift anomalies and discuss ways to keep your shift "out of the ditch" when one occurs.

Finally, as you develop your shift organization for the day, we show you how to prioritize patient care according to your overall patient assignment, individual patient needs, and other needs of the unit. Learning to prioritize at the bedside will also help you on tests and other demonstrations of your capabilities, including NCLEX-RN, annual skills sessions, and certifying examinations. We include examples of challenging prioritization test questions and provide answers with rationales.

Pre-Shift Planning

As you may have noticed in clinical rotations, your shift may actually begin before its scheduled time. This pre-shift time promotes a smooth transition, or hand-off, between shifts. Plan to be on your unit 20 to 30 minutes before your shift starts, according to your own comfort level and the approval of your nurse manager. A trend on units is not to allow early arrival. The objection is that when nurses clock in early, they create liability issues and increase payroll costs. Talk it over with those who set this kind of policy and see if they will allow you to arrive early if you will clock in at the designated time. Then set an alarm on your watch or cell phone as a reminder to clock in.

Consider asking the unit secretary or a departing RN how things went, and set an immediate intention to achieve desired outcomes on your own shift. In any event, arriving in time to make sure you have supplies and equipment needed, on your person or at the nurses' station, will set the right tone for the shift and give you a sense of control and organization. On many units, checking the medication administration system may be done in the middle of the shift, but you can add it to a list of things to do when feeling caught up and helpful. Begin by assisting your teammates:

- Perform safeguards related to narcotics, such as locating keys and completing the count or verifying the inventory in a locked system such as a medication administration system.
- Complete all resuscitation or crash-cart counts and any restocking assigned to Nursing.

- Answer phones or call lights.
- Restock IV fluids and supplies.

Contribute to a cohesive unit. Give the charge nurse time to evaluate patient acuity, consider staffing strengths and weaknesses, and complete assignments. The charge nurse will seek to start the shift on time and match patient acuity to the abilities of the staff scheduled for the shift. Manage your energy: come to work well rested, well fed, and with a positive attitude. Experiment with simple approaches that foster excellent working relationships:

- Smile! This free gesture is contagious and instantly corrects the sluggishness occasionally seen even at the start of a shift.
- Compliment a teammate. Feeling good is also contagious and lightens everyone's load.
- Offer to be a shift buddy for a teammate with a heavier assignment. Reciprocation typically follows.
- Bring fresh fruit or vegetables for the break room once or twice a season. Some teammates will catch on and bring something to share in a different season.
- Share solicitations for continuing education offerings that intrigue you. Your teammates will see you as a leader in pursuit of excellence.

Shift Report

Attend to the shift report and hand-off of patient care on your unit. You have no doubt noticed variability among different facilities and even on different units within one facility. You may have heard a taped report or experienced a verbal report "on the run." Or you may have received a verbal report in the nurses' station, report room, or at the patient's bedside. During orientation, ask about, observe, and participate with your preceptor to acquaint yourself with how nurses give report on your unit.

Be aware of a national movement for bedside reporting. This kind of face-to-face report addresses the Joint Commission's National Patient Safety Goal 13, a safety strategy that encourages the patient's active involvement in care. Bedside reporting also promotes effective communication, which is National Patient Safety Goal 2. This goal directly links to the issue of communication during report in three ways by:

- Targeting the need for concise, yet thorough, communication during patient hand-offs.
- Improving the effectiveness of communication among nurses.
- Allowing nurses and patients the opportunity to ask and respond to questions during hand-offs.

A structured communication technique such as I-SBAR-R provides a framework that streamlines information exchanges and promotes patient safety.

Once you know the style of report expected on your unit, decide what you need to know to organize your day and care for your patients. Adopt a shift organizer, which we refer to as "our brains" for the day. We include three sample shift organizers in Figures 6–1, 6–2, and 6–3 for you to try out or adapt to make your own. You may prefer a tool used by your preceptor, unit, or facility or even a blank sheet of paper. The key is to develop a system that is unique to how you think about and plan patient care. Systematic use of the same form every shift will further assist you to develop a smooth, organized, and safe plan of care for every patient assignment.

During report, use your shift organizer and fill in the blanks. Obtain HIPAA-approved information, including *patient age, allergies, room number, admission diagnosis, admitting provider, and resuscitation status*. Then obtain the following planning and assessment data, either through report or the electronic medical record (EMR):

- Intake and output (I&O) for the last shift
- Vital signs (VS) and heart rhythm
- Last time and dose of PRN pain and anxiety medication
- Relevant past medical history (PMHx)
- Current head-to-toe assessment
- Drains and dressings
- Relevant diagnostics, including procedures scheduled on or off the unit
- Recent change in condition
- IV sites
- IV fluids, rate, and amount hanging (credit)
- Ambulatory status
- Diet ordered
- Family dynamics
- "Psychosocial vital signs"
- Other needs

By the end of report, your goal is to "hit the ground running." A disorganized or insufficient report could require more time than is available to catch up on a patient's needs.

COACH CONSULT: FINE-TUNING A SHIFT REPORT

Just as starting IVs and dropping nasogastric (NG) tubes are skills to learn, so are listening to and giving reports. Whether giving or receiving report, think about what a novice nurse or float nurse would want to know about your patients. *Ask for too much* information at first. Over time and with role modeling from preceptors and other nurses, you will learn to ask for less as you become aware of alternative resources for information. *Give too much* information at first. You will learn quickly to give less based on the receiving RN's cues.

Room #			Room #		
Age	Sex	Spirituality needs	Age	Sex	Spirituality needs
MD		Phone	MD		Phone
Dx			Dx		
Allergies			Allergies		
Diet: NPO CL Bland DB Card Soft Thk REG Supl TF			Diet: NPO CL Bland DB Card Soft Thk REG Supl TF		
IVF	Rate	Site/Date	IVF	Rate	Site/Date
O's/Drains/Tubes:			O's/Drains/Tubes:		
Activity: Bed Dangle Commode BRP Chair Amb x ___			Activity: Bed Dangle Commode BRP Chair Amb x ___		
Bath: Self Bed Tub Shower Sitz Other			Bath: Self Bed Tub Shower Sitz Other		
I&O:	Time	Amount	I&O:	Time	Amount
I&O:	Time	Amount	I&O:	Time	Amount
I&O:	Time	Amount	I&O:	Time	Amount
I&O:	Time	Amount	I&O:	Time	Amount
BM	Flatus	Bowel Sounds x___	BM	Flatus	Bowel Sounds x___
Neuro			Neuro		
HEENT			HEENT		
Card			Card		
Circ			Circ		
Integ			Integ		
M/S			M/S		
Resp			Resp		
GI			GI		
GU			GU		
VS: T P R POx BP			VS: T P R POx BP		
VS: T P R POx BP			VS: T P R POx BP		
VS: T P R POx BP			VS: T P R POx BP		
Lab results: Gluc Na$^+$ K$^+$ Ca^{++}			Lab results: Gluc Na$^+$ K$^+$ Ca^{++}		
Other:			Other:		
Tests:			Tests:		
Other report:			Other report:		
0800			0800		
0900			0900		
1000			1000		
1100			1100		
1200			1200		
1300			1300		
1400			1400		
1500			1500		
1600			1600		
1700			1700		
1800			1800		
1900			1900		

F I G U R E   6 – 1 : Sample shift organizer for four patients (front and back).

Room #	Age Service Dx/Chief c/o	Report	VS Call H.O. Wt	Bowel Bladder I&O	Safety Activity Diet	O₂ Resp. Care	Tubes Drains Wounds	IV access Fluids Rates	Pain PCA	Teaching DC Plan	Labs	Known Drug Allergies
			FSBG p.ox. q8 q4 T> SBP> DBP> HR> RR> Sats< UO< ∨ ∨ ∨ ∨	I&O	SCD / REG CL FL NPO	ISq1hWA		CL: PIV: IVF:				
			FSBG p.ox. q8 q4 T> SBP> DBP> HR> RR> Sats< UO< ∨ ∨ ∨ ∨	I&O	SCD / REG CL FL NPO	ISq1hWA		CL: PIV: IVF:				
			FSBG p.ox. q8 q4 T> SBP> DBP> HR> RR> Sats< UO< ∨ ∨ ∨ ∨	I&O	SCD / REG CL FL NPO	ISq1hWA		CL: PIV: IVF:				
			FSBG p.ox. q8 q4 T> SBP> DBP> HR> RR> Sats< UO< ∨ ∨ ∨ ∨	I&O	SCD / REG CL FL NPO	ISq1hWA		CL: PIV: IVF:				

FIGURE 6–2A: Sample shift organizer for four patients (front).

RN:

DATE:

Room	**0800**	0900	1000	1100	1200	1300	**I&O 1400**	1500	1600	1700	1800
							I&O ___				
							I&O ___				
							I&O ___				
							I&O ___				

10:00: check & record lab values, do acuity sheets, record 4 hr. PCA totals; **14:00:** clear pumps, record I&Os, record 4 hr. PCA totals, update Care Plans & Goals, update charge nurse; **18:30:** all meds signed out?, replace MIVF bags so won't run out during shift change, record 4 hr. PCA totals, 12 hr. chart checks.

F I G U R E   6 – 2 B : Sample shift organizer for four patients (back).

Room #:			Physician:		Dx:		
Allergies					Hx:		
WBC 4.1-11.0	Platelets 140-400	Mg 1.5-2.5		AST 2-50		pH 7.35-7.45	
RBC 4.32-6.06	Sodium 135-145	Phosphorus 2.5-4.5		ALT 2-60		PCO$_2$ 35-45	
HGB 13.4-18.0	K+ 3.5-5.0	Chloride 98-110		BUN 7-25		PaO$_2$ 80-100	
Hct 40-54	Calcium 8.5-10.4	CO$_2$ 22-26		Creat 0.5-1.4		HCO$_3$ 23-26	

Time	Assessment	Body Diagram
1900 IV: PO: Rect:	Neuro: A/O Sedated Other_____	
2000 IV: PO: Rect:	Head/Neck: Eyes: Ears: Mouth: Nose:	
2100 IV: PO: Rect:	Respiratory/Vent: RUL____RML____ RLL____ LUL____ LLL____ Vent Settings: Wean: O$_2$:	
2200 IV: PO: Rect:	Tele/Cardiac: SR SB ST Afib IoAV BBB PVC PAC Paced	
2300 IV: PO: Rect:	GI: Bowel Sounds: Hypo Hyper WNL Absent NG: Nare: R L PEG:	
2400 IV: PO: Rect:	GU: Foley Rectal Tube Color: I/O _____ IN _____ OUT Last BM:	
0100 IV: PO: Rect:	Periphery: Arms: Pulses R/L WNL Absent Legs: Pulses D-R/L P-R/L WNL Absent Restraints: Flowtrons:	
0200 IV: PO: Rect:	Skin: D/I Moist Compromised Other: Edema: Anasarca:	
0300 IV: PO: Rect:	Vitals: TMax _____ SPO$_2$: _____ BP: _____ HR: _____ WT: _____	
0400 IV: PO: Rect:	Accu Checks: AC/HS Q6 BID	New Orders to Implement:
0500 IV: PO: Rect:	Diet: As tolerated NPO Cardiac Renal Diabetic Other_____ Tube Feed: Goal: Activity:	IV Access/Lines: TLSC: PIV: Gauge: CVP: Swan: Other:
0600 IV: PO: Rect:	AM Labs/Procedures CBC K Other: Chem 7 EKG Other: Mg C-XR Other: Phos Other:	Fluids Hanging/Med Drips: Maintenance: Sedation: Pressors: Other:
0700 IV: PO: Rect:	Test Results	Dressing Changes:

FIGURE 6–3: ICU shift organizer.

Conquering Shift Organization

To organize your shift, we recommend the IPAD mnemonic, detailed here and condensed in the margin note:

- *I*dentify: Begin with the end in mind. Identify shift goals and desired patient outcomes via available data. Apply what you learn during report from charts, medication administration records (MARs), and care plans. Use your shift organizer to promote a consistent approach to patient-centered care.
- *P*rioritize: Put your critical thinking skills to work. Review the section on prioritization, presented later in this chapter, to explore how use of the standards of the nursing process will increase your abilities and confidence to prioritize and reprioritize throughout any shift.
- *A*nticipate: Go beyond critical thinking to predictive thinking. Review available data for as-needed medications, ambulation orders, and diagnostic procedures. Ask the charge nurse for an update on expected discharges and admissions. Make a mental note of empty beds or divert status for unexpected admissions.
- *D*elegate: Add creative thinking to keep pace and manage your workload. Even if your unit does not employ assistive personnel, consider available resources at the beginning of each shift. If your team lacks patient care assistants, LPNs, or certified nursing assistants, consider negotiating with a charge nurse, team lead, or other RNs for mutually agreed-on delegation.

EVIDENCE FOR PRACTICE: ORGANIZING MY SHIFT

Use the IPAD mnemonic:
 *I*dentify
 *P*rioritize
 *A*nticipate
 *D*elegate

The IPAD method transforms the assessments and interventions required by your individual patients into a road map for implementation and evaluation of your entire patient assignment, including admissions, transfers, discharges, and trips off your unit for diagnostics and treatments. Decide during report the overall organization of patient care throughout your shift for both individual patients and your total group of assigned patients. Along with the information received in report, add the following activities to your planning:

- Preparation for discharge, which begins at admission.
- Possible times for patient and family teaching.
- Time to chart.
- Time for a meal and breaks.

Also include the tasks you plan to delegate and to whom. Remind yourself with a notation on your shift organizer to follow up on what you delegate. This comprehensive approach will allow you to regain some organization when you have a shift or patient anomaly. In addition, you will increase your chances of successful delegation if you make yourself available to teammates when your workload permits you to offer help. At the very least, negotiate with a fellow RN to be shift buddies. When you work with someone on a regular basis, you can communicate quickly when your buddy walks by. Be ready to delegate a specific activity.

PEAK PERFORMANCE: DELEGATION

Delegation is the process of transferring a selected nursing task to another individual who is competent to perform that specific task. Of critical importance, RNs may *not* delegate assessments to unlicensed assistive personnel. For example, when you ask a certified nursing assistant (CNA) to bathe patients, you may not delegate patient skin assessment to the CNA.

What is a shift or patient anomaly? We all have experienced them but may not have known this term. An anomaly is an irregularity, or something that deviates from the norm. Many anomalies occur in patient care. Box 6–1 lists commonly occurring patient anomalies.

Box 6-1 Commonly Occurring Patient Anomalies

- Patient falls
- Change in condition (your patient or another patient on the unit)
- Patient complaint/family complaint
- Patient discharged (beginning or end of shift or not expected)
- Patient admission (beginning or end of shift or not expected)
- Patient transfer to another unit (beginning or end of shift or not expected)
- Patient leaving against medical advice (AMA)
- Patient preparation for unexpected procedure
- Patient dies (your patient or another patient on the unit)
- Concern expressed by a colleague as to correct patient care
- Bedside procedure at beginning or end of shift

Sometimes more than one anomaly occurs within one shift. Although no one can anticipate every anomaly, maintain a high degree of suspicion. Consider the mechanism of injury or extent of deviation from normal limits. Anomalies are common in the following scenarios:

- A patient transferring from the operating room (OR) with a core temperature lower than 96°F may experience cardiac dysrhythmias.
- A patient who sustained a high-speed or head-on motor vehicle collision or who was unrestrained during a crash may have a bruised heart or lungs or both and experience mild to severe sequelae, including cardiac dysrhythmias or dyspnea.
- A unit that is in disarray, whether because of carelessness or in the aftermath of a dying patient or resuscitation patient, may provoke complaints from patients' families.

Ask for help when an anomaly occurs. Your charge nurse, preceptor, or supervisor may help solve the problem or delegate care. You can recover from a disruption to your overall shift organization through these steps:

- Identify the anomaly quickly.
- Prioritize the anomaly within your patient assignment plan of care.
- Anticipate any further anomalies.
- Use the IPAD method and assistance from others to help you recover from an anomaly.

COACH CONSULT: WHEN AN ANOMALY IS A SENTINEL EVENT

The Joint Commission defines a sentinel event as an unexpected occurrence involving death or serious physical or psychological injury, or the risk thereof. Serious injury specifically includes loss of limb or function. The phrase, "or the risk thereof," includes any process variation for which a recurrence would carry a significant chance of a serious adverse outcome. Such events are called "sentinel" because they signal the need for immediate investigation and response. The term "Never Event" was introduced in 2001 by Ken Kizer, MD, former CEO of the National Quality Forum (NQF), in reference to egregious medical errors (e.g., wrong-site surgery). Over time, the list has been expanded to signify adverse events that are unambiguous (clearly identifiable and measurable), serious (resulting in death or significant disability), and usually preventable. The NQF initially defined 27 such events in 2002.

Continued

PEAK PERFORMANCE: PRIORITY SETTING

Tune up your "priority-setting engine" by working through the clinical reasoning and judgment needed for the following patient assignments:

Room 101: Ms. Murphy Sign, 42 y.o. female S/P laparoscopic cholecystectomy (1 day ago) to be discharged today

Room 102: Mr. Sam Adams, 30 y.o. male with acute pancreatitis (alcohol abuse)

Room 103: Mr. Jonathon Wintergreen, 87 y.o. male with confusion and suspected urosepsis

Room 104: Ms. Jennifer Staples, 23 y.o. morbidly obese female S/P gastric bypass

Room 105: Ms. Sugar Maple, 57 y.o. female with poorly controlled type 2 diabetes mellitus

What would happen to your shift organization and prioritization if any of the following anomalies should occur?

Ms. Sign is ready to leave at the beginning of your shift.

Mr. Wintergreen pulls out his urinary catheter, climbs over the side rails, and falls.

Ms. Sign develops a fever and chills, *and* Mr. Wintergreen falls, *and* Mr. Adams shows signs and symptoms of peritonitis, *and* Ms. Staples arrives on the unit with her PACU nurse eager to give you a postoperative report, *and* Ms. Maple decides to leave AMA.

How would you recover from these shift anomalies? See approaches and rationales in Box 6–2, "Handling Anomalies."

End of Shift

Now we have come to the end of your shift when you will transfer care to another member of your team. It is just as important to end your shift in an organized manner. This consciously competent approach will help your teammates start their shift in an organized manner. Consider the transition in this way: Your end of shift is their pre-shift.

Box 6–2 Handling Anomalies

There are many ways to prioritize individual patient care and the overall patient assignment. You may change your order or rank with additional information. This exercise is to get you to think critically about and identify, prioritize, anticipate, and delegate your way through patient or shift anomalies.

1. *Ms. Sign is ready to leave at the beginning of your shift:*

Even a patient about to be discharged can put you off track. You may be able to handle this anomaly if report goes smoothly and you obtain all the information you need. If you are a nursing student or a new graduate on orientation, you and your preceptor could "divide and conquer." You also could ask for help from the nurse on the previous shift caring for the patient, your charge nurse, any unlicensed assistive personnel, or even your other patients. After a brief assessment of each patient, you could say, "I will discharge a patient and come back with your 8 o'clock medications. If I am not back when your breakfast arrives, please put on your call light." Your patients likely will remain *patient* and even help keep you on track by signaling you that their breakfast has arrived. Ask for help, and then remember to reciprocate when you catch up.

2. *Mr. Wintergreen pulls out his urinary catheter, climbs over the side rails, and falls.*

Your first concern is your patient. Take the time to assess him fully. Look for any possible head injury, and ask the patient's physician to order a computed tomography (CT) scan of the head if you even suspect the patient hit his head. Think of the sequelae that could occur if the patient takes the blood-thinning drug Coumadin. Examine his body for bruising, especially near the hips and wrists. After completing your assessment, ask for help to transfer him back to bed, and then notify the physician, charge nurse, and nurse manager or supervisor. Notify family members as well. Complete any additional interventions as ordered (e.g., frequent VS, imaging or x-rays, and reinsertion of new urinary catheter).

3. *Ms. Sign develops a fever and chills, and Mr. Wintergreen falls, and Mr. Adams shows signs and symptoms of peritonitis, and Ms. Staples arrives on the unit with her PACU nurse eager to give you a postoperative report, and Ms. Maple decides to leave AMA.*

This chaotic scenario could happen. How would you handle it? You will need to ask for help! Unlicensed assistive personnel might be able to get new VS on Ms. Sign and transport her to radiology. Mr. Adams' physician is on the unit and planning to transfer him immediately to the intensive care unit (ICU). You will need to assess Mr. Adams, gather documentation, and ask another team member to pack up his belongings and go to the ICU. Give report to the ICU, and return to the unit. You find Mr. Wintergreen on the floor, and Ms. Staples' nurse needs to give you report. Ask another nurse, your preceptor or charge nurse, to take report. Assess Mr. Wintergreen, call his physician with your assessment and new set of

Continued

Box 6–2 **Handling Anomalies—cont'd**

VS, and send him for a CT scan of the head. Now your teammate tells you Ms. Maple wants to leave now. You wanted to check in on your new patient (Ms. Staples), but you see that the charge nurse is still with her. You go to see Ms. Maple and talk with her about her reasons to leave. She wants to leave because the physician will not let her receive a visit from her dog. Whether or not this is a priority to you, this is a priority to Ms. Maple. Her physician arrives, and you assure him the dog can visit if it is up-to-date on all vaccines and stays only a short time. Ms. Maple agrees to stay. You now go to Ms. Staples' room and get report on your new patient. She is stable and you leave to prepare 0800 medications.

In preparing to give report and end your shift, collect the data needed for the most up-to-date assessment of your patients for your teammates:

- Visit your patients one last time.
- Review and update your shift organizer, patient assessments, care plans, and MARs.
- Give verbal or taped report according to the unit or facility's protocol. Include the same kinds of information you received. (Review the important elements from the list presented in the section on Shift Report.)
- Assist with change-of-shift duties.
- Complete your charting.

To accelerate your progress in shift planning, use reflective thinking to review that day's shift report and patient hand-off as you return home:

- Did you learn later that the preceding RN omitted important information, such as a diagnostic test scheduled for your shift? Next time, use your shift organizer as a checklist during report and ask questions. Hold accountable RNs who rush or seem careless.
- Did you get a negative reaction because you gave too much detail? Next time, pointedly say that you are giving the detail you would like to receive, and then ask what the receiving RN would like to know.
- Were you frustrated when the preceding RN wondered why you wanted to know a patient's age? Next time, patiently say you were considering adding some developmental goals to the care plan.

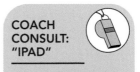

COACH CONSULT: "IPAD"

Review the IPAD mnemonic from time to time to tune up your shifting!

Prioritization

Prioritization puts a value on each assessment, intervention, or other activity and places them in rank order. This rank may relate to time or position with another activity. If something is a priority, it is a need or problem that requires immediate action. Translate "priority" with such words as "first, initial, immediate, most important, best, or safest." These words mean priority in both NCLEX-RN test questions and in actions at the bedside. Prioritize care of your patients using critical thinking and tools acquired in clinical rotations:

- Put your patients at the center of care. You and others on the interdisciplinary health-care team must mutually rank needs while considering patients' needs first.
- Review Box 6–3, "Prioritization Strategies," to keep the patient first and to address life-threatening versus non–life-threatening assessments.
- Prioritize other aspects of patient care according to integral theories of growth and development and implementation of care (e.g., Kubler-Ross theory of death and dying, Erikson's development theory, and teaching-learning theory).

PEAK PERFORMANCE: USING A THEORY TO SET CARE PRIORITIES

The classic Kubler-Ross theory of death and dying has mainstream acceptance, but its presentation suggests a simplistic linear progression that does not match reality. In 1995, Solari-Twadell et al. published the seminal pinwheel model of bereavement, which recognizes loss as a unique lived experience. Their pinwheel-shaped model—derived from research, theory, and clinical experience—captures the ebb and flow of grief and keeps the focus on the story of the deceased. Grieving family members resonate with this model and appreciate the way it honors their loved one through six core themes: being stopped, hurting, missing, holding, seeking, and valuing. Three larger themes of bereavement are change, expectations, and inexpressibility. The authors also identify nurses' capacities for "being with" the bereaved. Consider these themes when developing priorities in a plan of care for grieving family members. Your presence facilitates pattern recognition of family members' immediate needs. Your attentive listening initiates their search for words to begin expressing their grief.

Box 6–3 Prioritization Strategies

- Patient-centered (physical, psychological, safety, patient expectations)
- Life-threatening versus non–life-threatening
- Circulation, Airway, Breathing (CAB)
- Maslow's hierarchy of needs (physiological—survival, safety, and security; psychological—love and belonging; self-esteem; self-actualization)
- Growth and development theories (Erikson, Piaget, Freud, Skinner)
- The nursing process: assessment, diagnosis, outcomes identification, planning, implementation/intervention, evaluation (remember ADOPIE)
- Kubler-Ross' theory of death and dying: denial, anger, bargaining, depression, acceptance
- Teaching/learning theory

Look and act at the level of the patient by reviewing patient cases in the form of test questions that might appear on the NCLEX-RN or a certifying examination. Challenge yourself to think through this common clinical situation:

- What should the nurse do to meet the *patient's basic physical needs?*
  1. Pull the curtain.
  2. Answer the call bell immediately.
  3. Administer physical hygiene.
  4. Check VS.

Of course, all of these actions are important. To select the correct answer, think carefully about what the question asks. In this case, the question asks about the patient. The correct answer is option 3, which gives priority to administering physical hygiene, a *basic physical need* of the patient. Notice that the word "physical" is in both the stem of the question (what is being asked) and the correct answer. However, many test writers construct questions and answers to avoid such "giveaway" clues. Look for the principle being tested, and use a process of elimination.

Pulling the curtain and answering the call light immediately are important activities of staff on the unit, but they are not *basic care needs* of the patient. The word "immediately" creates a sense of urgency but does not alter the activity to a patient's basic physical need. Checking VS is important *to the nurse* and is one task completed during care of the patient. *Think patient first! What would he or she want?*

Now, examine a serious clinical situation:

- Your patient is asking you for a laxative as she has not had a bowel movement (BM) in 13 days. Her physician admitted her this morning with abdominal pain, vomiting, and dehydration. Her NG tube is putting out moderate amounts of brownish fecal material. She will have surgery at 4 p m. today. What would you do to provide the *best* care?
  1. Give her a laxative.
  2. Get an order for a laxative.
  3. Help the patient take her own laxative.
  4. Explain to the patient it is risky to give her a laxative at this time until the cause of her abdominal pain is determined.

As you may have surmised, this patient likely has a bowel obstruction. If the RN gives a laxative and stimulates peristalsis, a perforation of the bowel could result. The correct answer is option 4. In fact, the RN must *not* give a laxative. Instead, the RN should assess the patient's readiness for preoperative education, to include why the patient cannot receive a laxative; how to turn, cough, and deep breathe; and how to splint over the abdominal incision after her scheduled surgery.

Review the following scenario to prioritize nursing actions using the ABCs:

- Mr. Smith comes to the emergency department (ED) with an asthma attack. While trying to get to the ED, he trips and cuts his knee on some glass. What would you do *immediately?*
  1. Clean his knee, and prepare for suturing.
  2. Move his car for him as he parked in a no-parking zone.
  3. Administer oxygen and nebulizer medications.
  4. Measure his height and weight.

You likely know the correct answer is option 3. This patient needs his airway and breathing stabilized first before the cut in his knee receives care. What if you wondered further about ranking these activities? You would administer oxygen and an albuterol nebulizer to open his airways and supply his brain and body with oxygen. Once his oxygenation improves, you would obtain VS, including weight in anticipation of accurate dosing of any additional medications. Next you would clean his knee and assess for the likelihood of needing a suture tray. Finally, you would notify security about his car.

Maslow's hierarchy of needs—a model that demonstrates the biological, emotional, and psychosocial aspects of human needs and functioning—helps the RN establish priority actions related to human needs. A patient must attain one level of needs (physiological) before achieving the next higher level (safety and security):

- Physiological needs (necessary for survival, including pain management): First level
- Safety and security: Second level
- Love and belonging: Third level
- Self-esteem: Fourth level
- Self-actualization: Fifth level
- Aesthetic (larger meaning of life): Sixth level (sometimes included in the model)

Consider the following question:

- What should the nurse do to help meet a patient's *self-esteem needs?*
  1. Encourage the patient to perform self-care when able.
  2. Suggest the family visit the patient more often to complete all his care for him.
  3. Anticipate all needs before the patient requests help.
  4. Assist the patient with bathing and grooming only.

Option 1 is correct; the RN must encourage patients to meet their own needs to promote their self-esteem. The family may help but not complete all care. Options 2, 3, and 4 include the words "all" and "only." Those words are clues that the answer, especially on an NCLEX-RN question, is not correct. Words that mean "no exception" include "always," "never," "all," "every," "none," "must," and "only." Try not to use them on the unit, which will assist in your critical thinking at the bedside. Rarely is a situation "all or nothing."

Try two more questions using Maslow's hierarchy to prioritize among options:

- When administering oral medication to children, the *most important* factor to consider is their:
  1. Age.
  2. Weight.
  3. Level of activity.
  4. Developmental stage.
- A patient adaptation that may *initially* indicate internal abdominal bleeding postoperatively would be:
  1. Pain in the area of bleeding and an increased urinary output.
  2. Cool, clammy skin and a decreased heart rate.
  3. Restlessness and an increased heart rate.
  4. Hunger and a decreased urinary output.

For the first question, you would calculate the amount of any children's medication using a child's weight in kilograms (option 2). In adults, you would sometimes use weight but more often look at liver and kidney function to determine a safe dose of a medication. The second question requires you to know the differences between early and late signs of hypovolemic shock. If blood flow is reduced, the patient becomes restless and, as BP drops, the heart rate compensates and begins to increase (option 3). Late signs of shock involve a decrease in urinary output and eventually in cardiac output.

An example of caring for patients using developmental theories follows:

- In Erikson's theory of psychosocial development of the life cycle, which stage does the infant proceed through *first?*
  1. Identity versus role confusion
  2. Industry versus inferiority
  3. Initiative versus guilt
  4. Trust versus mistrust

The correct answer is option 4. This question requires you to recall the stages of development defined by Erikson. These stages are helpful to you at the bedside as you determine reasons for assessed or anticipated patient behaviors.

The standards of the nursing process also facilitate prioritization. Look at the following question:

- While on rounds, you find a patient on the floor in the hall. What should be your *immediate* response?
  1. Inspect the patient for injury.
  2. Transfer the patient back to bed so no one sees he or she fell.
  3. Move the patient to the closest chair.
  4. Report the incident to the nurse manager.

The first standard of the nursing process is assessment, so you would *assess* the patient first before moving him or her. Words related to assessment include "inspect," "auscultate," "percuss," and "palpate." Once you assess the patient, you can get help to return the patient to bed safely and then notify the physician, charge nurse, or nurse manager. You will also notify the family. Other staff on the unit can help watch the patient while you document the occurrence.

To determine a nursing diagnosis, whether at the bedside or for a test question, assess the patient first. Your assessment findings will guide you in deciding on the diagnosis. The following question is an example of using the nursing process to arrive at a priority nursing diagnosis:

- Your patient is 3 days postoperative. He reports pain of 2 to 3 on a scale of 10. His VS are stable, and he does not require oxygen.

He is taking clear and soft foods. He has not had a stool since surgery. The *most important* nursing diagnosis related to the information is:

1. Pain
2. Ineffective airway clearance
3. Sleep disturbance
4. Constipation

Typically, constipation (correct answer is option 4) would not be a priority nursing diagnosis, but if your assessment shows stability among other priority-setting strategies (e.g., ABCs), there is no better answer. The patient needs to increase fluids, increase ambulation, and receive a stool softener or laxative. This nursing diagnosis would be of priority on the patient's nursing care plan.

Another typical question or bedside assessment deals with the evaluation of a patient after receiving various treatments:

- You are evaluating Mr. Jones after administering medications for pain, bronchoconstriction, and low blood pressure. You are also looking for his lost wallet. Which of the following *outcomes* is *most important?*
  1. No c/o SOB, RR 18, regular
  2. Found wallet in pants pocket
  3. BP 120/70, HR 68, no syncope
  4. Pain 2/10

Using prioritization strategies, the ABCs apply, and option 1 is the correct answer. All actions are important, but when prioritizing a question or at the bedside, be most concerned about reducing bronchoconstriction to optimize oxygenation.

Consider this final question that is relevant to your daily clinical patient teaching. This question deals with teaching/learning theories and the importance of evaluating your patient's readiness to learn and his or her cognitive level:

- Which is *most important* when predicting the success of a teaching program regarding learning a skill?
  1. Only the learner's cognitive ability
  2. The amount of reinforcement after the program
  3. Only the extent of family support
  4. The interest of the learner

The correct answer (option 4) should stand out clearly from the rest of the possible answers. Note the word "only" in two of the answers. Words that signal "no exception" are a clue to an incorrect response. The amount of program reinforcement is not as important as the patient's readiness to learn. You will have nothing to reinforce if the patient is not ready to learn.

Chapter Summary

Conquering shift organization, giving and receiving report, and learning how to prioritize care are skills you will develop in your clinical practice. Remember to include the pre-shift time in your day, and be consistent in your setup of the day and delivery of report. Prioritize individual patients and your overall patient assignment using tools such as IPAD, patient-centered care, ABCs, and pertinent biological and psychosocial theories of care. Use the IPAD method to identify an anomaly quickly, prioritize immediate care, anticipate other anomalies that may follow, and delegate while asking for help. Critically reflect on "good" and "bad" shifts, "good" and "bad" reports, and "good" and "bad" hand-offs so that you may learn from them. Grab your keys—you are ready to go!

7 Communication: Mastering Collaboration, Delegation, and Documentation

CHAPTER 7

Communication: Mastering Collaboration, Delegation, and Documentation

The profession of nursing uses the nursing process to:
- Diagnose and treat human response to actual or potential health problems.
- Provide anticipatory guidance related to health, illness, and developmental stages across the life span.
- Promote health.
- Prevent disease.

Many nurses begin their careers in acute care settings at the bedside, where the first two above-listed professional aspects are paramount. The latter two aspects have more prominence in community health settings. Nurses in advanced practice address all four aspects in the course of a patient encounter.

In any health-care setting, the ability to convey a patient's response and maintain an effective nursing plan of care requires timely, efficient, and clear communication. This communication occurs between the nurse and other nurses, the patient, the patient's family, and others on the interprofessional health-care team. Additionally, communication typically requires written, verbal, and nonverbal components and assessment through evaluation of the patient's response to care.

This chapter features essential content related to communication:

- The importance of impeccable communication in the health-care setting.
- The guidance needed for exemplary interprofessional collaboration via appreciation of work styles across generations.
- The professional communication technique of I-SBAR-R (Introductions-Situation-Background-Assessment-Response-Readback).
- The principles of delegation along with its relationship to accurate and timely communication.
- The skill of documentation.

Communication

To communicate in any health-care setting, you must be able to gather and share competent information with patients, family members, physicians, other nurses, and the rest of the interprofessional team. This process involves sending and receiving messages that are verbal, nonverbal, and a combination of both. Often, the combination of communication methods clarifies the communication process more thoroughly than either method alone. Nurses use processes of communication to:

- Conduct a focused history and physical examination.
- Provide patient and family education.
- Give and receive report.
- Facilitate and delegate care among the interprofessional health-care team.
- Address changing patient conditions.

Effective communication is on the list of imperatives for every nursing curriculum, professional nursing organization, and health-care accrediting body. The second goal of the Joint Commission National Patient Safety Goals (NPSG) is to improve the effectiveness of communication among caregivers. Developing the knowledge, skills, and attitudes to promote effective communication is essential to your practice and to safe patient-centered care. The QSEN Institute makes the role of communication explicit among its competencies, especially related to teamwork, collaboration, and informatics.

Intraprofessional communication is a hot topic in nursing. More recent studies have shed light on two related phenomena: horizontal violence and generational differences among nurses. Walrafen et al. (2012) found most staff nurse participants stated they had witnessed or experienced eight of the nine behaviors associated with nurses' horizontal violence in their workplace. Sparks (2012) found significant differences between psychological empowerment scores for baby boomer and Generation X nurses, which could provide insight into inconsistent findings related to nurse job satisfaction. Sherman (2006) identified four generations of nurses in the work force: veterans (born between 1925 and 1945), baby boomers (born between 1946 and 1964), Generation X (born between 1965 and 1980), and millennials (born between 1981 and 2000).

To ensure the person with whom you communicate receives the same message you intend to send, study the process of nonverbal communication. Many factors influence the recipient's interpretation of your communication. Nurses include carefully selected, culturally sensitive nonverbal messages, which may result in a more accurate interpretation of a communication than a verbal message alone. Nonverbal messages include:

- Vocal cues, such as inflection, tone, intensity, or speed.
- Action cues, such as smiles, hand gestures, movement, and other forms of body language.
- Object cues, such as some physical piece of a routine that represents that routine, such as a bath basin for personal hygiene or a medicine cup for scheduled medication.
- Personal space cues, such as proximity when focus is needed or distance farther than 3 feet from a patient when you must leave a stable patient's room to attend to a more critical patient.
- Touch cues, such as an attention-getting hand to the shoulder or a comforting hand to the forearm.

If your vocal cues do not match your words, the recipient may not respond to *what* is said, but rather to *how* something is said. This mismatch can result in misinterpreting your meaning. For example, if your speech is calm, slow, reassuring, and without inflections that reflect disapproval, your patient will perceive the desired intent and be reassured. However, if your speech is rapid, loud, quivering, stammering, or condescending while you try to reassure a patient, your patient will recognize your uncertainty or judgmental position.

Although some professionals believe they may reach a particular audience through "street talk," in our experience this kind of short-term connection ultimately harms the rightful expectation of a professional encounter. To convey medical information to a layperson, you may need to explain terms in more common, everyday language or through the use of analogies or metaphors. For example, some patients or their family members would not know that the term "myocardial infarction" means heart attack. Medical jargon is essential to communicating with other members of the health-care team. Interprofessional jargon provides clarity and brevity among individuals communicating and produces an efficient form of report.

▲ PEAK PERFORMANCE: BIOCOMMUNICATION

In October 2012, during a keynote address at the 39th Annual National Conference on Professional Nursing Education and Development, Kristen Swanson, PhD, RN, FAAN, Dean, University of North Carolina Chapel Hill, distinguished among biocommunication styles first described by Halldorsdottir about 20 years earlier. All biocommunication styles are identified in the following list, but only biogenic and bioactive styles potentiate what Swanson termed nursing's *healing trinity*: caring, safety, and leadership. How discerning and intentional are you in the way you communicate with patients and members of the health-care team?

- Biogenic or life-giving communication that promotes healing: "I feel honored to be your nurse. The goals you set today for participating in your care are inspiring and mark a path to your well-being."
- Bioactive or life-sustaining communication that is concerned, compassionate, and competent: "I'm interested in your thoughts and feelings before the surgery ... Here is the equipment that will drain away excess fluid so you will heal more quickly. Tell me more about your fear of going home with drains still in place."
- Biopassive or life-neutral communication that is detached or disengaged: "Your surgery is routine. Your surgeon will explain the approach. If you have any more questions, I will return just before your surgery to answer them."
- Biostatic or life-restraining communication that is blind to others' plight or even neglectful of others because they are a nuisance: "Read this brochure about your surgery. It explains everything and answers frequently asked questions."
- Biocidic or life-destroying communication that is acid-edged, alienating, or diminishing: "I have three other patients who are sick, and I'm really busy with their needs. I don't have time to explain JP drains to you. Besides, it's no big deal to go home with a drain in place."

PEAK PERFORMANCE: ASSESSING CUES

The following case example demonstrates what can happen if the message sent is not the message received.

A 70-year-old Asian-American woman was admitted to your medical-surgical unit for complaints of "a little stomachache." She explains she has experienced pain in her abdomen for the past 3 days. She states her daughter insisted on bringing her to the emergency department. As you document her admission history and physical examination, you notice she winces when changing position, holds her abdomen while leaning forward in the chair, is pale and diaphoretic, and has dry mucous membranes. Additionally, she reports vomiting several times today and having her last bowel movement 1 week ago. She describes her abdominal pain as "a little achy" and rates it as 3 out of 10. She states she does not want to bother anyone and should just go home.

Do the verbal and nonverbal cues for pain match?

Is this patient likely sicker than she describes?

It is apparent that the verbal and nonverbal cues observed with this patient do not match. She states her pain is merely achy (scored 3 out of 10), but the observed physical assessment suggests to you she is in considerably greater pain (winces when changing position, holds her abdomen while leaning forward in the chair, and is pale and diaphoretic).

The patient likely is quite ill, as she exhibits the observed findings and reports vomiting several times today with her last bowel movement 1 week ago. A patient her age and with her signs and symptoms may be experiencing a small bowel obstruction, which can be a life-threatening pathophysiological problem.

Understanding that people of different ages, cultures, backgrounds, and personality types receive and interpret the same communication differently is essential to effective communication. For example, if you tell a patient and family members that the patient's urinary output is less than 15 mL per hour, they may not receive this information the same way as a physician, advanced practice nurse, or staff nurse on the unit. Similarly, if a patient declines admission to the hospital for lifesaving treatment because no one is at home to feed the cat, you must receive this communication with the intended sincerity and urgency of the message.

Different cultural communication patterns also need consideration. For example, the volume of speech of a European American, African American, or Arab American may be louder naturally, and a Chinese American may misinterpret this volume as a sign of anger. Therefore, nurses must listen with twice the intensity as they speak. The late business leader Stephen Covey put the maxim this way: We must seek first to understand those we are communicating with before we can be understood.

One cut-to-the-chase method for effective communication comes via our Coach Quadrants, depicted in Figure 7-1.

- The upper right quadrant represents the ideal: AO stands for "appropriate observation," which you deliver with an "I" message. Appropriate observations begin with phrases such as "I noticed," "I am curious," and the nonjudgmental "I wonder." Whatever follows comes from your own perspective, leaving you accountable for the words that complete the sentence.

- The upper left quadrant is valuable when needed: AC stands for "appropriate critique," which you deliver with an "I" message in private. An appropriate critique registers a complaint without judgment or personal criticism, and the person issuing the complaint is in a position of authority to do so. The context for authority varies in health-care settings, but the ideal is a collaborative environment in which every voice brings value to safe, competent, and principle-centered patient care. We must also empower patients with the authority to issue a complaint related to their subjective experience.

- The lower left quadrant is not therapeutic. IO stands for "inappropriate observation," which reflects a communication style that puts patients on the defensive. This style is recognizable because it begins with "you," as in "You have not gotten

WINDOW ON COMMUNICATION STYLES

AC	AO
IO	IC

FIGURE 7–1: Coach Quadrant: Window on communication styles.

out of bed today." Even more problematically, "you" messages often result from exasperation and carry the additional mistake of exaggeration ("you always" or "you never"), as in "You always put on your call light within 5 minutes after I leave your room."

- The lower right quadrant represents unprofessional behavior. IC stands for "inappropriate critique," which often manifests as public criticism. Turn on your systems thinking and gauge the climate on your unit: Is public criticism at the nursing station a common occurrence? You can make a difference in the professional tone on your unit when you make a suggestion about an unprofessional interaction, such as "Please take this conversation into the conference room."

To confront a patient's problematic or puzzling behavior, consider using ICE questions. The ICE mnemonic refers to progressive statements that address behavior typically labeled as "noncompliant." We prefer to regard this kind of behavior as nonadherent and seek a patient's underlying belief. ICE stands for:

- *I = Interest:* Statements of interest help when nonadherent behavior first surfaces: "I am interested in you and your life. Tell me about the challenges you're facing because of your diagnosis."

- *C = Curiosity:* Statements of curiosity may reveal a persistent obstacle: "I am curious about your routine for taking your medications."

- *E = Explanation:* Statements seeking explanation may offer insight into unhealthy behavior: "I wonder if you can explain your request for food choices that are not on the prescribed menu." Notice the insertion of "I wonder," which softens the use of "you." You can soften the statement further by using "describe" instead of explain. This approach offers an appropriate way to explore a patient's accountability without damaging the relationship.

COACH CONSULT

Nurses must maintain a therapeutic relationship with their patients. A powerful rationale comes from Covey's business text, *Seven Habits of Highly Effective People,* in which he referred to inflicted relationship damage as making a withdrawal from the recipient's emotional bank account. Patients often have so little reserve that nurses will have no opportunity for patient education if they inflict this sort of damage under the guise of paternalistic "patient compliance."

Whether you are completing a focused or comprehensive assessment, you will use the techniques of a patient interview, including cues from patient observation, and findings from your physical assessment to gather and interpret information. This information, together with the nursing process and your increasing clinical judgment, facilitates your development of mutually agreed-on goals and an appropriate nursing plan of care.

The patient interview is a structured communication with the purpose of obtaining subjective data from the patient. The patient interview requires the use of interpersonal communication skills in which you maintain a neutral, nonjudgmental position. A competent approach to interviewing features three systematic parts:

- **Introduction phase.** Many nurses walk in and "get busy," forgetting to introduce themselves to the patient. This gaffe hinders the establishment of rapport. Introduce yourself, and give your patient the opportunity to ask any immediate questions. Preoccupied patients will have difficulty focusing on *your* questions.
- **Working or data collection phase.** Subjective data derive from the patient's health history and the patient's current experience. Patients' thoughts, beliefs, feelings, sensations, and perceptions of a problem are their current symptoms. Subjective data include anything the patient says. Symptoms are not objectively measurable and may come from the patient (primary source), a family member (secondary source), or, if necessary, previous medical records (secondary source). You may ask both open and closed questions as you gather subjective information.
- **Termination phase.** This phase features three parts. First, you will give an overview of the next several hours to days, according to what you already know about the patient's situation. Second, you and the patient will set some mutual goals. Third, you will begin planning for discharge. Most units have a formalized approach with preprinted forms to complete and route to ancillary services such as a social worker or home health agency.

This consistent approach paves the way for a smoothly conducted patient interview, promotes development of an interpersonal connection, and facilitates pattern recognition on behalf of patients' safety and well-being. Patterns also include an array of pitfalls (see Box 7–1, "Potential Pitfalls of the Patient Interview Process"). When you recognize yourself in the midst of a pitfall, correct the error, and restate your question: "I just asked you two questions at once. Let me ask them one at a time."

Box 7–1 Potential Pitfalls of the Patient Interview Process

- Leading the patient: "You look better today. You must be feeling better."
- Limited objectivity because of bias: "My own father was an alcoholic, too."
- Letting family members answer for the patient: "The mother always says the patient has a headache."
- Asking more than one question at a time: "Have you had a bowel movement and walked around the unit today?"
- Not giving time for the patient to respond to the question: "What do you understand about your surgery today? Let me just give you this brochure."
- Using medical jargon: "Since you had an MI, your CABG times 4 is set for tomorrow."
- Assuming or jumping to conclusions: "Great job! You ate all of your lunch" (when, in fact, the patient's son ate it).
- Taking a patient's comments personally: "I don't want to stay in the hospital. I want to die." (You did not cause the patient's wish.)
- Offering false reassurance: "You've got the best surgeon in the country."
- Giving advice: "The best way I found to stop smoking is with a nicotine patch."

During the interview and the physical assessment, you collect data as you observe your patient. Initial observations provide clues to both overt and covert problems and assist in prioritizing your physical examination. Engage your critical thinking further by using senses that increase your efficiency. For example, when you take a blood pressure, feel the patient's skin for temperature and turgor, smell his or her general body odor (fruity breath raises suspicion for high blood glucose or diabetic ketoacidosis), listen for any audible breathing (wheezes could signal respiratory tract obstruction), and see overt grimacing. Other sense-dependent questions might include:

- While observing your patients, do they appear ill or in distress?
- What are they doing while you observe them? Are their nonverbal cues consistent with their verbal communication?
- Have you observed any unusual movements? For example, clonus in a pregnant woman suggests pre-eclampsia.

Once you have developed a personal connection with your patient, completed the patient interview, and noted your observations, perform the physical examination. To promote the relationship needed for mutual goal setting, communicate what you do, why you do it, and what you find. An

COACH CONSULT

What communication techniques facilitate a successful patient interview?

- Acknowledge a patient's response.
- Use silence effectively.
- Clarify if you are unsure of a response.
- Restate the patient's main ideas.
- Be an active listener.
- Use reflection, redirection, focusing, and sequencing to prevent misinterpretation.
- Use judicious humor to reduce anxiety.
- Summarize what you heard, and give your patient an opportunity to correct your summary.

engaged patient will facilitate your ability to hone in on normal and abnormal findings. In general, you will inspect, palpate, percuss, and auscultate (IPPA) each body system warranting investigation. If you assess the abdomen, however, the order will be inspect, auscultate, percuss, and palpate so as not to alter bowel sounds before auscultation.

Communication of your findings is one of your most important roles. Communication during a shift report or when delegating a task must be clear, concise, and complete, consisting of correct and up-to-date information. Think through what you will say, using your shift organizer to promote this careful approach. For example:

- You do not want to report to the next shift that your patient last had IM morphine 6 hours ago when you just discontinued the parenteral morphine and administered oral narcotic analgesics.
- Similarly, you do not want to delegate the task of assisting with a patient's meal if the patient's status will shortly change to NPO (nothing by mouth).

In Chapter 6, we reviewed important information to communicate during report. Later in this chapter we will review communication during delegation, including the Five Rights of Delegation.

Now we explore coach quadrants related to work styles that affect communication. Many of us have experienced a communication event in which conflict occurred; for example, when two or more physicians or advanced practice nurses prescribed for different interests or goals. Conflict can occur as you communicate with many different people each shift and in stressful or emergent situations. Perspectives may be different but are usually not right or wrong. Participants in a potential conflict can reframe their positions by collaborating or compromising. Figure 7–2 depicts the coach quadrants related to work styles:

- **Collaboration** represents the ideal work style because solutions are win-win. Collaborative communication initially may take more time but actually saves time in the long run by preventing drawn-out review of conflict.

WINDOW ON WORK STYLES

Compromise	Collaboration
Accommodation	Conflict

FIGURE 7-2: Coach Quadrant: Window on work styles.

- **Compromise** is an acceptable work style because each party wins some and loses some. Compromise is particularly effective among peers.
- **Accommodation** is less desirable, although common, because one party gives in, resulting in a lose-win outcome. Accommodation is the stereotypical nursing work style, which is correctable through empowerment and competent negotiation and collaboration.
- **Conflict** is unprofessional because both parties lose "face" and respect. Conflict also requires energy to repair the damage. How much better to put that amount of energy toward collaboration or compromise!

COMMUNICATION

Why is communication important? People crave communication! In some studies, not to mention stereotypical perceptions, most people believe women speak more than men. Yet, Mehl et al. (2007) found that both genders speak on average about 16,000 words per day.

If you encounter conflict and are uncertain how to handle it, ask for help from your charge nurse or nurse manager. Many situations can be resolved through compromise, in which parties agree to disagree with one another while focusing on what is best for the patient.

I-SBAR-R

Communicating effectively with others on the interprofessional health-care team is essential for quality patient care and patient safety. It is of

COACH CONSULT

Cultural humility is a crucial perspective in professional nursing and encompasses another essential element of communication: to meet health-care expectations for patients with limited English proficiency. Although being multilingual imparts a valuable advantage, any nurse can recognize and respond to needs for accurate translation and interpretation that minimize dependence on unreliable or inappropriate substitutes, such as patients' relatives or friends.

In fact, using family members as interpreters can defeat our efforts to provide patient education. A former student told us, "I was trying to explain to a Spanish-speaking patient why he might choose Tylenol over ibuprofen, depending on his liver and kidney function. As I listened to the adult son interpret, I realized he used the Spanish word for stomach in each instance of kidney or liver."

The Patient Protection and Affordable Care Act of 2010 reauthorized the Office of Minority Health to help eliminate health disparities among racial and ethnic minority populations

Continued

Box 7-2 Common Phrases and Questions in Three Languages

ENGLISH	SPANISH	FRENCH
Good morning.	Buenos días.	Bonjour.
My name is _____.	Me llamo _____.	Je m'appelle _____.
I am a nurse.	Soy enfermero/ enfermera.	Je suis infirmière.
What is your name?	¿Cómo se llama?	Quel est votre nom?
How old are you?	¿Cuántos años tiene?	Quel age avez-vous?
Show me ...	Enséñeme ...	Montrez-moi ...
Here There	Aquí Allí	Ici Là
Which side?	¿En qué lado?	Quel côté?
Right	Derecha	A droite
Left	Izquierda	A guache
How long?	¿Cuánto tiempo?	Combien de temps

particular importance in the event of a patient's changing condition. The Institute for Health Care Improvement and the Joint Commission endorse the quality and safety communication technique called SBAR (pronounced "ess-bar"), which stands for *S*ituation, *B*ackground, *A*ssessment, and *R*esponse. Numerous hospitals as well as the military and some airlines use this system to facilitate rapid, accurate communication among team members (Fig. 7–3).

SBAR is an easy communication method that is useful for framing any routine for critical interprofessional health-care conversation. The situation (*S*) is the current problem or reason for communicating with the health-care provider. The background (*B*) provides important elements from the patient's past or current medical history and physical examination. The assessment (*A*) is the nurse's assessment of the situation. The response (*R*) shares recommendations for patient-centered, evidence-based, quality care.

Grbach (2007) and the QSEN Institute made recommendations to strengthen the original SBAR communication and to support the Joint Commission NPSG related to communication among health-care workers. A new acronym, I-SBAR-R, was developed, in which *I* = *Introduce* (self and patient) and *R* = *read back* (orders). Compare results between haphazard communication and I-SBAR-R in the following scenarios.

Example: Non–I-SBAR-R:

"This is Sheila calling about Ms. Smith. She's now putting out 400 mL of blood-tinged discharge per hour from her NG tube. Her heart rate is a little higher than it has been. Her temperature is stable. I'm not sure what her BP is. I think she had labs drawn this morning, but I can't find the chart. She just doesn't look good to me." The physician gave orders and the nurse replied, "OK, I'll get these done and call back later."

Analysis Using Critical Thinking:

    I: Introduction: Was it complete?

    S: Situation: Was it complete? What changed?

    B: Background: When was this patient admitted? When did she have surgery?

    A: Assessment: What other information did the physician need?

    R: Response: Do you know what the physician said?

    R: Read back: Did the nurse read back any orders to the physician?

Same Example: Using I-SBAR-R:

"Hello, Dr. Winter, this is staff nurse Sheila Jones from University Center Hospital on the surgical unit. I am calling about Ms. Sara Smith whom you admitted 48 hours ago. She has put out 400 mL of blood-tinged

COACH CONSULT —cont'd

through policy and program development. One such effort is National Standards on "Culturally and Linguistically Appropriate Services," commonly referred to as the CLAS document. Standards related to removing communication barriers address culturally competent care, language access services, and organizational supports for cultural competence.

Nurses can promote rapport with non–English speaking patients by initiating conversations in prevalent languages spoken in their geographic areas. Box 7–2, "Common Phrases and Questions in Three Languages," lists 10 common phrases and questions in English, Spanish, and French. Many more phrases and medical terms are included in "The Interpreter in Three Languages," an appendix of *Taber's Cyclopedic Medical Dictionary* (Newland, 2013; Venes, 2013).

SBAR report to physician about a critical situation

S	**Situation**
	I am calling about <patient's name and location>
	The patient's code status is <code status>
	The problem I am calling about is _____.
	    I am afraid the patient is going to arrest.
	
	I have just assessed the patient personally:
	
	Vital signs are: Blood pressure ____/____, Pulse____, Respiration____, and Temperature____
	
	I am concerned about the:
	    Blood pressure because it is over 200 or less than 100 or 30 mm Hg below usual
	    Pulse because it is over 140 or less than 50
	    Respiration because it is less than 5 or over 40
	    Temperature because it is less than 96 or over 104

B	**Background**
	The patient's mental status is:
	    Alert and oriented to person, place, and time
	    Confused and cooperative or non-cooperative
	    Agitated or combative
	    Lethargic but conversant and able to swallow
	    Stuporous and not talking clearly and possibly not able to swallow
	    Comatose. Eyes closed. Not responding to stimulation.
	
	The skin is:
	    Warm and dry
	    Pale
	    Mottled
	    Diaphoretic
	    Extremities are cold
	    Extremities are warm
	
	The patient is not or is on oxygen.
	    The patient has been on _____ (L/min) or (%) oxygen for_____ minutes (hours)
	    The oximeter is reading ____%
	    The oximeter does not detect a good pulse and is giving erratic readings

A	**Assessment**
	    This is what I think the problem is: <say what you think is the problem>
	    The problem seems to be cardiac infection neurologic respiratory_____
	    I am not sure what the problem is but the patient is deteriorating.
	    The patient seems to be unstable and may get worse; we need to do something.

R	**Recommendation**
	I suggest or request that you <say what you would like to see done>.
	    Transfer the patient to critical care.
	    Come to see the patient at this time.
	    Talk to the patient or family about code status.
	    Ask the on-call family practice resident to see the patient now.
	    Ask for a consultant to see the patient now.
	Are any tests needed:
	    Do you need any tests like CXR, ABG, EKG, CBC, or BMP?
	    Other?
	If a change in treatment is ordered, then ask:
	    How often do you want vital signs?
	    How long do you expect this problem will last?
	    If the patient does not get better, when would you want us to call again?

FIGURE 7–3: SBAR handout.

discharge over the last 4 hours from her NG tube. She is 24 hours post-op colon resection and had put out a total of 400 mL bile-colored drainage from her NG tube in the first 20 hours. Her heart rate is up to 116 bpm from 90 and her BP is down to 90/60 mm Hg from 130/76. I would like to draw a stat CBC, type and crossmatch, and obtain an abdominal CT." *(Dr. Winter gives Nurse Jones orders.)* "OK, Dr. Winter, I will order a stat CBC, type and crossmatch for 2 units packed RBCs, and an abdominal CT. I will call you with the results as soon as they are available."

Analysis Using Critical Thinking:

> I: *Introduction:* Was it complete?
>
> S: *Situation:* Was it complete? What changed?
>
> B: *Background:* When was this patient admitted? When did she have surgery?
>
> A: *Assessment:* What other information did the physician need?
>
> R: *Response:* Do you know what the physician said?
>
> R: *Read back:* Did the nurse read back any orders to the physician?

The use of this standardized communication ("hand-off technique") will become second-nature to you after some practice. Each item of the I-SBAR-R communication will help you report the situation more accurately and facilitate the physician or advanced practice nurse to make safe, high-quality health-care decisions.

EVIDENCE FOR PRACTICE

Since endorsing the use of SBAR in 2006, the Joint Commission has published a study of this communication technique in a multihospital system. Findings showed SBAR was generally well understood; 97% of the nurses who participated in the study had been educated about SBAR. Challenges included inconsistent uptake across facilities, lack of physician education about SBAR, and a tendency to view SBAR as a document rather than a verbal technique (Marill, 2013).

Delegation

Delegation is the process of working with and by means of another member of the health-care team to complete patient care. The National Council of State Boards of Nursing defines delegation as the transfer of a specific nursing task, in a specific situation, by a nurse to another competent health-care provider. As this definition also states, the nurse delegating the task remains accountable for the completion, evaluation, and documentation of that task. In addition, as the nurse learns the art of delegation, he or she begins with the patient's preferred outcomes in mind.

The Five Rights of Delegation are helpful. The rights are (1) the right circumstance with (2) the right task assigned to (3) the right health-care provider using (4) the right direction (clear, concise, correct, complete communication), with (5) the right supervision. An RN can delegate only some daily tasks performed in patient care. The RN cannot delegate aspects of the nursing process, clinical judgments, or interventions that require professional nursing knowledge, judgment, or skill (counseling, patient/family education, skills outside the provider's scope of practice). The RN must reassess delegated tasks during a shift when a patient's condition changes.

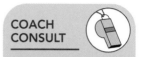

COACH CONSULT

Delegation is a key aspect of leadership. Delegation allows you to make the best use of your time and skills, and it helps other people on the health-care team grow and develop to reach their full potential.

Documentation

Nearly every encounter with a patient requires documentation. Accrediting bodies, state licensing laws, and your state's nurse practice act legally mandate a nurse's documentation of the following:

- Communication with patients, families, and health-care providers.
- Outcomes of the nursing process: after every assessment, implementation of an intervention, evaluation of an intervention, and patient education session.
- Delegation and follow-up of tasks.

Problem-oriented medical records (POMRs) provide all members of the health-care team a way to document their involvement in patient care. Many facilities use standard forms, computer records, checklists, or charting by exception. Whatever is the standard for your unit is the documentation format you will use to communicate effectively. Becoming familiar with the guidelines of documentation is essential to your safe and legal practice. The four C's of communication will help you communicate effectively:

1. Clear
2. Concise

3. Correct
4. Complete

Every health-care agency maintains policies and procedures related to documentation. Some facilities still document on paper, whereas many others have converted to electronic health records (EHRs), which are sometimes called electronic medical records (EMRs). Many patient charts continue to use source-oriented documentation, with each profession completing different sections of the chart. Other facilities use POMRs, on which anyone on the interprofessional health-care team involved in the patient's care charts in the same section and on the same progress notes. This method provides a sequencing of events or care provided to the patient regardless of who provides the care.

Several tools are available for documenting and communicating your findings.

- SOAPIE: S = subjective data, O = objective data, A = assessment or nursing diagnosis, P = plan to affect the human response to this health problem, I = intervention used, E = evaluation of the effectiveness of the intervention and resolution of a nursing diagnosis.
- PIE: An abbreviated version of SOAPIE: P = problem or nursing diagnosis, I = intervention, E = evaluation completed by the nurse.
- DAR: D = data; A = action, or the intervention used to affect the problem; and R = response, similar to an evaluation of the action or intervention.
- CBE = charting by exception, which some facilities use with focused or narrative charting for abnormal findings; checklists document normal and abnormal findings, and the nurse explains abnormal findings more thoroughly in a narrative form in the progress or nurse's note.

Regardless of the documentation method, the following guidelines apply:

- Verify you have the correct chart before you begin documenting.
- If writing, use black ink, and write legibly. If typing, use correct spelling.
- Date and time every entry and every page without skipping lines or leaving blanks. (EHR systems will automatically record date and time.)
- Use objective, factual, complete documentation; avoid judgmental statements.

- Document care, medications, treatments, or procedures as soon after their completion as possible. Do *not* document in advance— perhaps you may leave the unit before giving a medication, key equipment breaks down, or a procedure is canceled.
- Document the patient response to all interventions.
- Document consent or refusal of treatment.
- Document telephone calls, messages, and orders.
- Sign your name and title with each entry, although automatically added with EHR.
- Use quotations as appropriate in subjective data.
- Follow your agency's policy for late entries and errors. In general, nurses cross out any errors with one line, to prevent obliterating an entry, and date and initial the correction.
- Use correct spelling, punctuation, and grammar.
- Use only abbreviations accepted by your unit or facility, and keep up to date with the Joint Commission's official list of "do not use" abbreviations.
- Maintain privacy and confidentiality of documented information.

ALERT

Have you heard the phrase, "If it isn't documented, it wasn't done"? Courts of law have upheld this statement. For example, if you say you assessed a patient's toes for color, movement, and sensation, yet the patient's cast was constricting blood flow and the patient lost his or her foot, a court can find you responsible if you did not document your findings.

CLINICAL VOICE: INTERPROFESSIONAL COMMUNICATION

The importance of interprofessional communication comes to light in the following case study.

I was working as a charge nurse on a medical/surgical unit when notified that a patient was being admitted from the PACU s/p vaginal hysterectomy. The patient was coming to our unit because the gynecology floor was full. We were told she was an 18-year-old who had had an uneventful PACU course. I assigned her to a very experienced LPN for her care while I would complete her post-op admission assessment and hang any IV fluids. The patient was brought to the unit accompanied by her mother.

The hallway report explained that the 18-year-old woman was deaf and could not speak. Her VS had been stable throughout her stay in the PACU. Her surgeon would visit her in the morning. Her mother translated using sign

> ### CLINICAL VOICE: INTERPROFESSIONAL COMMUNICATION—cont'd
>
> language that she was tired and wanted to sleep. I completed an assessment and left her with the LPN and CNA to complete VS every 15 minutes.
>
> Over the next hour, the patient's blood pressure slowly dropped, and her heart rate slowly increased. She remained sleeping but easily aroused. She had no vaginal discharge and no additional urine output. Her mother was no longer in the room with her, so I sent another staff member to look for her. I had a bad feeling that something was wrong and worried she was bleeding internally. I assigned a CNA to remain with the patient and to continue to measure her VS every 15 minutes. I gathered my facts and paged the surgeon.
>
> The surgeon called back and listened to my concerns. She said she had an office full of patients and could not come to see the patient. As I hung up the phone, the LPN returned to say the patient's VS were worsening, and I quickly went to assess the patient. Her VS were now: BP 80/40, pulse 126 bpm, and respirations shallow at 26. We placed her in a Trendelenburg position, and I called the surgeon and my nurse manager. My nurse manager arrived as I completed the call with the surgeon. Again, the surgeon stated she could not come to see the patient. She gave no new orders. After a brief conversation and another set of VS, the decision was made to move up the "chain of command." The chief of surgery happened to respond, came to assess the patient, ordered 2 units of packed RBCs, and transferred her to the ICU. She went to surgery, where more than 1 L of blood was found in her pelvis. A "bleeder" was cauterized, and the patient recovered without incident.
>
> That day I learned how much we need our communication skills to communicate effectively with our colleagues. I realized, after debriefing with my nurse manager, that I did not say specifically to the surgeon, "I need you to come and see your patient now. If not, I will follow up the chain of command." If I had communicated more effectively, I could have enlisted help sooner. Thankfully, the patient received the care needed and did not suffer any negative outcomes.

Chapter Summary

The nursing skills of communicating, delegating, and documenting are as important to learn as starting an IV, ambulating a patient, or completing a sterile dressing change. The technique of I-SBAR-R supports the four C's of communication (clear, concise, correct, and complete) in relating a change in patient condition to a physician, advanced practice nurse, or other member of the health-care team. Communication in delegation supports safe, quality, patient-centered care when the delegating nurse clearly explains the tasks and provides timely follow-up and documentation.

8 Critical Nursing Actions: Responding to Key Situations

CHAPTER 8

Critical Nursing Actions: Responding to Key Situations

A patient's progress toward attainment of desired outcomes is the focus of the American Nurses Association (ANA) Standards of Care regarding nursing assessment, diagnosis, outcome identification, plan, implementation, and evaluation. These familiar standards constitute the nursing process and its component parts. This chapter focuses on three *critical* nursing actions:

1. Responding to changing patient conditions.
2. Managing pain.
3. Providing end-of-life care.

Attention to these areas not only will accelerate your practice from novice to advanced beginner to competent nurse, but such attention also will make you stand out among your peers. Agencies consistently report shortcomings among nurses for these nursing actions in their first few years of practice.

We first describe what to do in the process of a changing patient condition and reinforce the use of I-SBAR-R, introduced in Chapter 7, to communicate assessments. We focus next on advanced strategies for managing patients' acute and chronic pain. In the last section, we address the less familiar but emerging territory of hospice, palliation, and end-of-life care of patients and their families.

Responding to Changing Patient Conditions

Essential to standards-driven communication is notifying physicians of changing patient conditions in accordance with National Patient Safety Goals. These goals focus on the problems identified in health-care safety and how to resolve them to improve patient safety. Guidelines for improving interprofessional communication cover the following important questions:

- When should the nurse notify a physician?
- What change in a patient's condition has occurred?
- What is the best way to communicate the change?

Beginning as a nursing student, you must communicate swiftly and accurately with your preceptor or clinical instructor. Your precepting nurse then communicates with the patient's attending physician, consulting specialists, residents, and family members to relay any change assessed in a patient. Reasons to contact a physician commonly occur with changes in the circulatory, neurological, respiratory, gastrointestinal, or musculoskeletal systems. Table 8–1, "Criteria for Notification of Patient Condition," lists some of the most important criteria for informing the physician when a patient experiences a change in condition. For example, it is important to notify the physician:

- If a patient's blood pressure (BP) changes from a baseline of 120/70 mm Hg to 90/50 mm Hg.
- If a patient who has been resting comfortably complains of chest pain and shortness of breath.
- If a patient can no longer move one or more extremities.

In Chapter 7 we introduced the situational communication model called I-SBAR-R for the members of an interprofessional health-care team. The following hypothetical example illustrates the use of I-SBAR-R in an acute change in a laboratory value and associated change in the patient's mental status:

> *I*ntroduction: "Hello, Dr. Summer, this is Charge Nurse Harry Jones from University Center Hospital's MICU. I am calling about Mr. Emmett Washington whom you admitted this morning."
>
> *S*ituation: "Mr. Washington's blood glucose at 1,100 was 500 mg/dL."
>
> *B*ackground: Mr. Washington is a 55-year-old black man admitted status post (s/p) acute myocardial infarction (AMI). He has a history of coronary artery disease (CAD), hypertension (HTN), dyslipidemia, and type 2 diabetes mellitus (DM).

Table 5-1 Criteria for Notification of Patient Condition

CIRCULATORY SYSTEM	Unexplained decrease or increase in BP or in baseline heart rate (HR)	Sustained decrease in urine output (UO) <30 mL/hr	Uncontrolled hemorrhage	New-onset cardiopulmonary (CP) or acute electrocardiogram (ECG) changes
NEUROLOGICAL SYSTEM	Change in level of consciousness (LOC), speech, alertness, sensation, movement	Acute change in Glasgow Coma Scale	New-onset or uncontrolled seizures	
RESPIRATORY SYSTEM	Decreased oxygen (O_2) saturation requiring increase in O_2 (i.e., from nasal cannula [NC] to mask)	Acute change in chest tube drainage or bubbling	Acute changes in breath sounds or in respiratory rate or pattern	
GASTROINTESTINAL SYSTEM	Blood in emesis or stool	Sustained decrease (>2 hr) in UO <30 mL/hr	Acute abdominal distention, uncontrolled vomiting	Increasing complaint of (c/o) abdominal pain
MUSCULOSKELETAL SYSTEM	Color, movement, sensation check indicating lack of pulses, cool extremities, acute swelling, change in sensation	Sudden inability to move or weakness of extremity		

Continued

Table 5–1 Criteria for Notification of Patient Condition—cont'd

OTHER: MEDICATIONS AND REACTIONS	Drug reaction	Medication error or blood transfusion reaction		Any laboratory result reported as "critical value"
ACUTE LABORATORY TEST CHANGES	Blood sugar (BS), activated partial thromboplastin time (aPTT), prothrombin/international normalized ratio (PT/INR)	White blood cells (WBCs), hemoglobin and hematocrit (H&H) levels	Potassium (K^+), magnesium (Mg), calcium (Ca^{++})	
METABOLIC	Acute change in temperature; BS			
SURGICAL	Dehiscence of wound or evisceration of organs	New or increasing wound erythema	Worsening circulation, motion, or sensation signs	
DISRUPTION OF TUBES	Clotting of central line access; dislodged surgical drainage device; nasogastric (NG), Dobhoff tube, etc., swelling or tenderness at insertion site	Change in peripherally inserted central catheter (PICC) line position or status, disruption of/change in position of chest tube		
PATIENT FALLS	Together with completion of incident/occurrence report			

Assessment: His vital signs (VS) are stable, but his blood glucose levels have increased from 237 mg/dL at 0700 to 320 mg/dL at 0900 to 500 mg/dL at 1,100 mg/dL. He is also lethargic. He is currently receiving a regular insulin intravenous (IV) drip at 2 U/hr.

Response/Recommendation: "I am concerned that the patient's blood glucose will continue to rise unless we increase his insulin dose."

Read back: (Dr. Summer gives Nurse Jones orders and . . .): "OK, Dr. Summer, I will write the order to increase the insulin drip to 5 units per hour and repeat a stat blood draw for glucose level in 2 hours. I will call you with the results as soon as they are available."

Analysis Using Critical Thinking:

I: Was it complete?

S: Was it complete? What changed?

B: When was this patient admitted? How rapidly did his blood glucose level increase?

A: What other information did the physician need?

R: Do you know what the physician said?

Read as many I-SBAR-R briefings as possible to accelerate your mastery of this patient safety communication technique and to improve your ability to respond confidently to changing patient conditions. The Web site of the QSEN Institute provides examples at www.qsen.org; other examples can be found in clinical nursing journals.

EVIDENCE FOR PRACTICE: WORSENING PATIENT CONDITION

Stress-induced hyperglycemia has been associated with poor outcomes and death in critically ill patients. Blood glucose (BG) variability, a component of stress-related hyperglycemia, has been reported more recently as a significant independent predictor of intensive care unit and hospital mortality. In 2011, Reed et al. conducted three case studies and found that although decreasing BG variability is an important aspect of hyperglycemia management, new-onset events of BG variability may be a sentinel warning or occur as a physiological response to a worsening patient condition. These events warrant rapid investigation and treatment of the underlying problem.

Managing Pain: Pathophysiology and Patient Care Strategies

Well-controlled pain is one of the most nurse-sensitive patient outcomes and a major contributor to patients' satisfaction with health-care delivery. Although many nursing textbooks refer to pain as the fifth vital sign, it is not a sign at all. Pain is a symptom that cannot be measured objectively. It is an unpleasant sensory or emotional experience associated with actual or potential tissue damage. Pain is also whatever a patient says it is. Health-care providers and patients themselves commonly undertreat pain, which can lead to chronic pain. Chronic pain alters the daily processes of life in all of these areas:

- Physiological
- Psychological
- Sociocultural
- Behavioral

Because of these far-reaching implications, it is essential to accelerate your understanding of the pathophysiology of pain and effective strategies for managing pain.

Pain occurs through the *transduction, transmission, perception,* and *modulation* of messages sent via the peripheral nervous system (PNS) and central nervous system (CNS). *Transduction* is the reception and transfer of the sensation called pain from the site of injury ultimately to the CNS. Nociceptors in tissues are stimulated by mechanical, thermal, or chemical injury and transmit information to the CNS. These nociceptors are in the skin, subcutaneous tissues, joints, artery walls, and internal organs and respond, via nerve signals, to various stimuli. Tissue trauma (mechanical stimulus), extreme cold or heat (thermal stimulus), or tissue ischemia (chemical stimulus) causes the release of cell breakdown products and inflammatory mediators. Any of these substances can activate nociceptors. The result is pain.

Once transduction of pain has occurred, *transmission* of pain to the spinal cord and brain follows unless inhibited (Fig. 8–1). The electrical conduction of pain transmits along two types of primary afferent nerve fibers, which carry impulses toward the spinal cord and brain. A-delta fibers transmit sharp, stabbing, or intermittent pain rapidly along the myelinated sheath of a nerve. C fibers are responsible for slow transmission of pain signals, resulting in constant, dull, aching pain. In response to a pain-inducing injury, afferent nerve fibers transmit impulses to the dorsal horn of the spinal cord. In the dorsal horn, transmission of pain

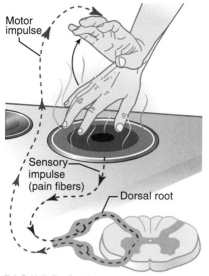

FIGURE 8-1: Pain transmission.

either continues on to the brain or is inhibited. Several substances either activate or inhibit further transmission. When nerve signals leave the spinal cord, they reach the thalamus, somatosensory cortex, limbic system, and frontal cortex of the brain. The patient perceives and interprets this electrical stimulus as pain (somatosensory cortex), experiences an emotional response to the pain (limbic system), and thinks about the cause of pain (frontal cortex).

Next, the patient becomes aware of, or *perceives,* pain. All humans possess the same *pain threshold,* or the point at which a stimulus is painful. However, everybody has different *pain tolerances.* Past experiences with pain and an individual's psychosocial and cultural makeup shape the individual's tolerance to pain (see Table 8–2, "Cultural and Ethnic Variations in Response to Pain").

Pain *modulation* and sensitization occur during the process of recognizing pain. Analgesia or competing pain stimuli can modulate or adjust the sensation of pain (Fig. 8–2). People become sensitive to pain from peripheral or central processes. Peripheral sensation to pain occurs as a result of prolonged exposure to a painful stimulus. As exposure continues,

Table 8–2 Cultural and Ethnic Variations in Response to Pain

CULTURAL GROUP	RESPONSE TO PAIN
African American	Pain is a sign of illness or disease. Absence of pain may affect compliance with treatment (i.e., may not take medication as prescribed unless pain present). Pain is considered inevitable and must be endured. Spiritual and religious beliefs account for high tolerance to pain. Persistent pain is associated with little faith. Prayer and laying on of hands are used to treat pain.
Appalachian	Pain is endured and accepted stoically. Believe use of objects can rid pain (e.g., knife or ax under the bed to "cut out" pain).
Arab American	Pain considered unpleasant and something to be controlled. Expression of pain less with strangers and more with family; send conflicting perceptions of pain. Confidence in Western medicine, expect immediate relief of pain.
Chinese American	Description of pain more diverse in terms of body symptoms, such as pain more dull and diffuse. Explain pain from the traditional influences of imbalances in *yin* and *yang*. Cope with pain using oils, massage, warmth, sleeping on affected area, relaxation, and aspirin.
Cuban American	Pain is a sign of physical problem that warrants traditional or biomedical healer. Response to pain very expressive (i.e., crying, moaning, groaning), considered a pain-relieving function.
Egyptian American	Avoid pain and seek prompt treatment. Expression of pain less with strangers and more with family; send conflicting perceptions of pain. Description of pain more generalized. Age and birth order correlate with individual responses and description of pain (e.g., younger children and first-born more expressive about pain). Helpful to have close family member present during pain episodes, preferably woman, who is seen as more nurturing, caring, and capable of comforting patient in pain.
Filipino American	Pain considered part of living an honorable life. Pain considered as means to atone for past transgressions and achieve fuller spiritual life. Response to pain stoic, tolerant of great amount of pain.

Table 8–2 Cultural and Ethnic Variations in Response to Pain—cont'd

CULTURAL GROUP	RESPONSE TO PAIN
	May need to encourage use of pain interventions. May use prayer in pain management.
French Canadian	Pain described as more intense; described more effectively.
Greek American	Pain (*ponos*) considered cardinal symptom of ill health. Pain considered evil and needs to be eradicated. Family relied on to find resources to relieve pain. Physical pain expressed publicly, but emotional pain kept within privacy of family.
Iranian	Expressive about pain. Men more stoic than women in expressing pain. May justify pain in light of later rewards after death.
Irish American	Stoic response to pain; may ignore or minimize pain. Denial of pain may delay treatment.
Jewish American	Preservation of life paramount; therefore seek immediate treatment for pain. Verbalization of pain is acceptable and common. Want relief from pain and to know cause.
Mexican American	Good health associated with being pain-free. Pain considered necessary part of life. Obligated to endure pain in performance of duties. Type and amount of pain divinely predetermined. Pain and suffering considered consequences of immoral behavior. Methods used to relieve pain maintain balance within person and environment. Perceptions of pain may delay seeking treatment.
Navajo Indian	Pain must be endured, leading to inadequate pain control. May use herbal medications to treat pain.
Vietnamese American	Pain is endured, considered part of life. Cultural restraints against showing weakness limit use of pain medication.

Purnell, L. & Paulanka, B. (2003). *Transcultural Health Care: A Culturally Competent Approach,* ed. 2. Philadelphia: F.A. Davis.

COACH CONSULT

Table 8–2, "Cultural and Ethnic Variations in Response to Pain," provides practical information about culture and pain that contributes to an efficient pain assessment. However, more recent perspectives would caution against the potential for stereotyping patients based on cultural aspects, which are ultimately context dependent. Ray (2010) uses the mnemonic *CARING* to address patients' needs, suffering, problems, and questions that arise in culturally dynamic situations:

Compassion
Advocacy
Respect
Interaction
Negotiation
Guidance

Ray further lists a more comprehensive approach to caring, culled from nursing literature and made memorable through the initial letter "C" for each of nine concepts to be considered in holistic care of any patient, particularly when a patient is experiencing pain:

- Compassion
- Competence

Continued

the patient's pain tolerance decreases, resulting in an increased response to pain (hyperalgesia) or a sensation of pain to a nonpainful stimulus (allodynia). Central sensitization to pain also occurs with prolonged exposure. Although the mechanisms of these types of sensitization differ, any of them may result in chronic pain.

It is important to understand the pathophysiological development of pain because pharmacotherapy is geared to alleviating pain at its many different physiological triggers or other processes. Pain is also treated nonpharmacologically according to the different types of pain. Table 8–3, "Types of Pain, Causes, and Treatment," lists the types of pain and causes, duration, effects on the patient, and examples of mechanical, thermal, or chemical stimulation that cause pain. Treatments vary depending on whether pain is acute, chronic, or malignant. Therefore, recognizing a patient's particular type of pain helps the health-care team plan for appropriate and responsive care.

In addition to a patient's self-report, the most important way to determine the type of pain is by recognizing its underlying pathophysiological cause. Two major divisions of pain are nociceptive and neuropathic pain. Nociceptive pain occurs with exposure to a mechanical, thermal, or chemical stimulus that produces tissue injury. It is a protective response to acute tissue damage. Nociceptive pain can manifest as visceral or somatic pain. Deep visceral pain occurs when an organ undergoes overdistention, traction, spasms, an ischemic event, or inflammation. Visceral pain may be localized or diffuse (hard to point to) or cause referred or radiating pain to sites other than the site where the pain originated. Referral or radiation of pain often occurs because of shared nerve pathways between different sites. Typically, the quality of visceral pain is aching to sharp and stabbing and may be accompanied by autonomic nervous system signs and symptoms, such as diaphoresis, nausea and vomiting, pallor, pupil dilation, tachycardia, tachypnea, increased blood pressure, and muscle tension. Somatic pain may originate in superficial or deep body structures. Superficial somatic pain originates in the

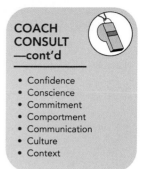

COACH CONSULT —cont'd

- Confidence
- Conscience
- Commitment
- Comportment
- Communication
- Culture
- Context

skin or mucous membranes. Patients often characterize this kind of pain as sharp or burning. Tenderness on palpation, along with hyperalgesia, hyperesthesia (increased sensitivity to sensory input or stimuli), and allodynia (such as in fibromyalgia), may occur. Deep somatic pain originates

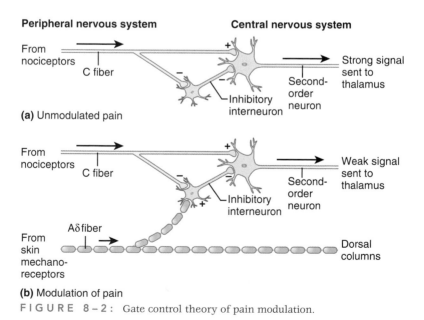

FIGURE 8–2: Gate control theory of pain modulation.

Table 8–3 Types of Pain, Causes, and Treatments

TYPES	CAUSES	TREATMENTS
Nociceptive—Mechanical	Arthritis, fractures, disk herniation, postsurgical, spinal stenosis, tension headache, muscle injury	NSAIDs, stretching, epidural or trigger-point steroid injections, surgery
Nociceptive—Chemical	Kidney or gallstones, cardiac ischemia or infarct, stomach ulcer, Crohn disease	Opioids, corticosteroids, surgical repair
Nociceptive—Thermal	Burns, frostbite	Opioids
Neuropathic	Diabetic neuropathy, postherpetic neuralgia, phantom limb pain, myofascial pain syndrome, disk herniation	Opioids, nerve-stabilizing agents (gabapentin, oxycarbazepine, zonisamide), epidural steroid injections, spinal blocks

in muscles, bones, and joints of the body. This type of pain can be localized, diffuse, or radiating and may be caused by injury, ischemia, or inflammation from acute or chronic injury.

Neuropathic pain occurs after injury to the PNS or CNS. This type of pain provides no protective mechanisms against further tissue injury and often becomes the disease itself. Categories of neuropathic pain include mononeuropathic/polyneuropathic pain, deafferentation pain, sympathetically maintained pain, and central pain. This type of pain is often chronic and debilitating.

EVIDENCE FOR PRACTICE

In the first edition of this textbook, we reported on an interprofessional group of researchers at Walter Reed Army Medical Center that studied the promising effects of mirror, or visual illusion, therapy involving patients with phantom limb pain after the amputation of a leg or foot (Chan et al., 2007). Several studies have appeared in the literature since then related to phantom limb pain, including a comprehensive review of mind-body interventions, such as hypnosis, imagery, biofeedback, and the visual mirror feedback reported in our first edition (Moura et al., 2012). Mechanisms of action for mind-body interventions target cortical reorganization, autonomic nervous system deregulation, stress management, coping ability, and quality of life. Related studies on meditation, yoga, and tai chi/qigong were missing from the literature.

Pain assessment is the cornerstone of pain control (see Chapter 3) and drives the cycle of the nursing process through intervention and evaluation of treatment effectiveness. This cycle includes a reassessment of pain characteristics and area of tissue injury. Current recommendations for reassessment of a patient include:

- Within 30 minutes after parenteral pain medications.
- Within 1 hour after oral pain medication.
- After any patient report of a change in pain level.

The following section focuses on advanced strategies for managing patients' acute and chronic pain. Regardless of cause, patient, or type of pain, every patient deserves adequate pain control through attention to the following aspects of care:

- Assessment—objective physical findings, subjective reports of pain, and complete physical assessment follow-up when findings are inconclusive.
- Mutually set goals for pain management.
- An interprofessional approach.
- Nonpharmacological and pharmacological treatments.
- Patient and family education about treatment modalities.
- Prevention of adverse effects.
- Evaluation of the effectiveness of all therapies.

Drug therapy for pain control, whether for acute or chronic pain, includes nonopioid analgesic agents, opioid analgesics, and co-analgesics. The World Health Organization (WHO) Analgesic Ladder (Fig. 8–3), which has demonstrated its effectiveness and widespread usefulness after more than 25 years of use, lists the various analgesic modalities for treatment of pain according to severity. An adaptation of this ladder has emerged for neurosurgical procedures. This model adds a fourth step, to include nerve block, epidurals, patient-controlled analgesia pump, neurolytic block therapy, and spinal stimulators (Vargas-Schaffer, 2010). Pain management also may include interventional therapies and nondrug therapies. We encourage you

WHO ANALGESIC (PAIN RELIEF) LADDER

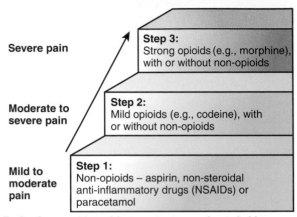

Severe pain

Step 3:
Strong opioids (e.g., morphine),
with or without non-opioids

**Moderate to
severe pain**

Step 2:
Mild opioids (e.g., codeine), with
or without non-opioids

**Mild to
moderate
pain**

Step 1:
Non-opioids – aspirin, non-steroidal
anti-inflammatory drugs (NSAIDs) or
paracetamol

F I G U R E 8 – 3 : World Health Organization analgesic ladder.

to take the lead in your workplace by learning as much as you can about safe and effective pain management and attending to commonly occurring barriers (see Box 8–1, "Barriers to Effective Patient Pain Management").

Nociceptive pain results from injury to skin, joint, muscle, or visceral tissue. It typically occurs from an acute injury and responds well to both nonsteroidal anti-inflammatory drugs (NSAIDs) and opioid analgesics. Mild to moderate pain, rated 1 to 4 out of 10, is treated with nonopioid analgesics such as aspirin, acetaminophen (paracetamol on the WHO Analgesic Ladder), or any of the classes of NSAIDs. Infrequently, oral or injected corticosteroids accompany pain management to help resolve inflammation. Nonpharmacological treatments include rest,

---

Box 8–1 Barriers to Effective Patient Pain Management

Barriers to pain management for health-care providers include the following:
- Lack of education
- Poor pain assessment skills
- Concerns over prescribing opioids (less than 1% of patients experience addiction)
- Concerns over respiratory depression as an adverse reaction
- Regulatory concerns

ice, compression, and elevation (RICE) and stretching (see Box 8–2, "Nonpharmacological Interventions for Pain Management").

More severe nociceptive pain, described by the patient as moderate to severe (rated 3 to 6 out of 10), likely will require both NSAIDs and moderate-strength opioid analgesics:

- Codeine.
- Hydrocodone (with acetaminophen [Norco, Vicodin, Lortab]).
- Oxycodone (with aspirin [Percodan], with acetaminophen [Percocet, Roxicet, Tylox]).
- Ketorolac.

For acute pain, nonpharmacological treatments such as RICE and stretching may help relieve pain. For chronic pain, additional interventions include massage, physical therapy, and epidural or trigger-point injections.

Severe nociceptive pain (rated 7 to 10 out of 10), as occurs with burns, trauma, and kidney stones or in the immediate postoperative period, requires strong opioids with or without nonopioid analgesics. Morphine is the gold standard for opioid analgesics. Other strong opioids include:

- Meperidine (Demerol) (*note:* refer to a current *Davis's Drug Guide* for safe administration of any drug, and this drug in particular).
- Methadone.
- Heroin.
- Fentanyl.
- Hydromorphone (Dilaudid).
- Oxymorphone.

Box 8–2 Nonpharmacological Interventions for Pain Management

- RICE
- Heat therapy
- Relaxation, biofeedback
- Massage, stretches
- Transcutaneous electrical nerve stimulation (TENS) unit
- Percutaneous electrical nerve stimulation (PENS) therapy
- Acupuncture, acupressure
- Hypnosis
- Distraction
- Brace, splint, cast
- Exercise
- Surgery

Severe acute pain is protective to a patient because the pain limits movement and allows for healing. Nonpharmacological treatments such as RICE, relaxation, and distraction also may be effective adjuncts to analgesics for severe acute pain.

Neuropathic pain results from damage to nerves in the PNS or CNS. Causes of neuropathic pain include trauma, inflammation, metabolic diseases, infections involving the nervous system, tumors, toxins, and neurological diseases (see also Table 8–3). This type of pain is not protective and can develop into chronic, poorly controlled, mild, moderate, or severe and persistent pain. Often, neuropathic pain does not respond well to opioid analgesics, and other medications and nonpharmacological treatments are necessary to provide the patient with pain relief. Box 8–3, "Co-Analgesic Drugs Used to Treat Neuropathic Pain," provides a list of drug classes used as co-analgesics. These agents work together with NSAIDs and opioids to enhance pain relief.

Box 8–2 presents other interventions used in patients with chronic pain. As a last resort, some patients and health-care providers elect surgical interventions in an attempt to resolve a patient's pain. New therapies are evolving to treat even the most difficult types of neuropathic pain (see Evidence for Practice).

EVIDENCE FOR PRACTICE

In patients with dementia, undertreatment of pain, particularly central neuropathic pain caused by white matter lesions, is widespread. A current review of the literature encouraged a combination of self-report pain rating scales (in particular, the Verbal Rating Scale, the Horizontal Visual Analogue Scale, or the Faces Pain Scale) and pain observation scales. Assessment of sensory abilities (e.g., touch, pinprick, temperature, vibration) and mood (e.g., anxiety) and determination of the presence of a Babinski reflex, accelerated tendon reflexes, and spasticity also may contribute to a reliable determination of pain. Next to pharmacotherapy, nonpharmacological treatment strategies such as transcutaneous electrical nerve stimulation (TENS) may be effective as long as afferent pathways transmitting the electrical stimulus are still intact.

Box 8–4, "Adverse Effects to Watch for in Patients Taking Opioid Analgesics," and Box 8–5, "Opioid Overdose: Signs and Symptoms and Treatment," present information related to adverse effects of opioid analgesics and opioid overdose, both of which need priority attention

---

Box 8-3 Co-Analgesic Drugs Used to Treat Neuropathic Pain

- Tricyclic antidepressants (amitriptyline)
- Selective serotonin reuptake inhibitors (SSRIs) (fluoxetine)
- Lidocaine patches
- Antiseizure medications (gabapentin [Neurontin], carbamazepine [Tegretol])
- Capsaicin
- Anesthesia/blocks

Box 8-4 Adverse Effects to Watch for in Patients Taking Opioid Analgesics

- Respiratory depression
- Constipation
- Orthostatic hypotension
- Urinary retention
- Biliary colic
- Cough suppression
- Emesis
- Increased intraocular pressure (IOP)
- Miosis
- Euphoria or dysphoria
- Sedation

Box 8-5 Opioid Overdose: Signs and Symptoms and Treatment

Classic triad of overdose:
- Coma
- Respiratory depression
- Pinpoint pupils

Treatment:
- Ventilatory support
- Opioid antagonist: naloxone (Narcan)

---

in the plan of care and patient education. Anticipation of unexpected events or anomalies promotes pattern recognition and prompt action in the event of their occurrence. The opioid antagonist naloxone (Narcan) reverses the signs and symptoms of opioid overdose and possibly saves the life of a patient who displays them. However, patients who receive this intervention also feel immediate pain. A new but altered course of analgesics needs to be secured as close to the administration of an opioid antagonist as possible.

Providing End-of-Life Care

In 1997, the Institute of Medicine reported on the need to improve end-of-life (EOL) care. That same year, the American Association of Colleges of Nursing and a group from the City of Hope National Medical Center came together to outline nursing competencies important in the provision of quality EOL care. These pioneers, called the End of Life Nursing Education Consortium (ELNEC), have educated thousands of nurses in quality EOL care according to the consensus document titled *A Peaceful Death: Recommended Competencies and Curriculum Guidelines for End-of-Life Care.* This document focuses on alleviating suffering and promoting comfort at the end of a patient's life.

Assessing patients for advance directives and EOL care wishes is as essential as asking patients about their past medical history or known allergies. However, many nurses have not acquired the knowledge, skills, and attitudes regarding advance directives and EOL care to attend fully to these important patient needs. In this section we clarify terms associated with palliative and EOL care (see Table 8–4, "Terminology Related to End-of-Life Care"). We also review the importance of maintaining patients' quality of life regardless of their disease, prognosis, or ability to pay. Next, we discuss in depth the use of palliative care in chronically ill

Table 8–4 Terminology Related to End-of-Life Care

TERMINOLOGY	DEFINITION	AUTHOR OF DEFINITION
Palliative care	Active total care of patients whose disease is not responsive to curative treatment. Prevent, relieve, reduce, or soothe the symptoms of disease or disorder without effecting a cure.	World Health Organization (WHO) Institute of Medicine (IOM)
End-of-life (EOL) care	Holistic care provided explicitly during the final weeks of life when death is imminent.	Ferrell and Coyle

Table 8–4 Terminology Related to End-of-Life Care—cont'd

TERMINOLOGY	DEFINITION	AUTHOR OF DEFINITION
Hospice care	Program of care that supports the patient and family through the dying process and the surviving family members through bereavement.	Hospice Foundation of America
Peri-death nursing care	Process of dying and death comprising a series of biological and emotional changes.	Matzo
Active dying	Process of total body system failure.	Pitorak
Prognosis	To determine the course that a disease may take from a point in time until death, including an understanding of the disease processes and trajectories and of end-stage indicators.	Matzo
Transition point	Event in the trajectory or course of an illness that moves a patient closer to death.	Matzo
Patient Self-Determination Act	Amendment to the Omnibus Budget Reconciliation Act of 1990; requires Medicare/Medicaid agencies that provide health care to notify patients they have the right to participate in and direct their own health-care decisions, accept or refuse medical or surgical treatment, prepare an advance directive, and receive information regarding the provider's policies that govern the utilization of these rights.	U.S. Congress
Patient Bill of Rights	Statement of the rights to which patients are entitled as recipients of medical care: information disclosure, choice of provider/	American Hospital Association

Continued

Table 8–4 Terminology Related to End-of-Life Care—cont'd

TERMINOLOGY	DEFINITION	AUTHOR OF DEFINITION
	plan, access to emergency services, participation in treatment decisions, respect and nondiscrimination, confidentiality, ability to appeal, consumer responsibilities.	
Dying Person's Bill of Rights	Be treated as a human being, maintain sense of hopefulness, express feelings, participate in care decisions, realize comfort goals, not to die alone, be free from pain, die in peace, have questions answered honestly, not be deceived, receive help for family, receive respect for body after death.	Southwestern Michigan Inservice Education Council Workshop
Allow Natural Death (AND) order	Type of advance directive that calls for a proactively based approach to end of life based on positively describing the contents of care, rather than focusing on the negative "do-not" directives.	Venneman et al., 2008
Do Not Resuscitate (DNR) order	Type of advance directive requesting not to receive cardiopulmonary resuscitation (CPR) in the event of a cardiopulmonary collapse.	American Academy of Family Physicians
Durable power of attorney for health care	Type of advance directive stating whom the patient has chosen to make health-care decisions in the event the patient cannot make his or her own medical decisions	American Academy of Family Physicians
Living will	Type of advance directive and legal document describing what medical or life-saving treatments the patient agrees to if he or she becomes seriously or terminally ill.	American Academy of Family Physicians

Table 8–4 Terminology Related to End-of-Life Care—cont'd

TERMINOLOGY	DEFINITION	AUTHOR OF DEFINITION
End-of-Life Nursing Education Consortium (ELNEC)	National curriculum that addresses the critical aspects of EOL care: palliative care, pain management, symptom management, ethical and legal response, cultural considerations, communication, grief, loss, bereavement, quality EOL care, and care at the time of death.	American Association of Colleges of Nursing and City of Hope National Medical Center
Medical Orders for Scope of Treatment (MOST) form	Type of advance directive adapted from the Physician Orders for Life-Sustaining Treatment (POLST) paradigm that began in Oregon in 1991. The MOST form is a bright pink provider (MD, DO, PA, or NP) order sheet, based on a person's medical condition and wishes. The form combines elements of the Five Wishes and a living will into one document that addresses CPR, medical interventions, antibiotics, medically administered fluids and nutrition, and a basis for the order, including a patient's or authorized representative's review and agreement.	Caprio et al., 2012
Thanatology	Study of death.	DeSpelder and Strickland

patients and explore a synopsis of the signs and symptoms of impending death and care to provide at the time of death. The chapter concludes with an overview of organ donation or procurement and care of the bereaved.

The Patient Self-Determination Act (PSDA) of 1990 obligated health-care providers to ask patients on admission to a health-care facility about their understanding of advance directives. Many patients and facilities have promoted patient self-determination in EOL care by means of the following directives:

- Do Not Resuscitate (DNR) order.
- Allow Natural Death (AND) order.
- Patient Bill of Rights.
- Durable power of attorney for health care.
- Living will, Five Wishes, or Medical Orders for Scope of Treatment (MOST) form.
- Dying Patient's Bill of Rights.

LEADING CAUSES OF DEATH IN AMERICANS IN 2011

1. Diseases of the heart
2. Malignant neoplasms (cancer)
3. Chronic lower respiratory diseases
4. Cerebrovascular diseases
5. Accidents (unintentional injuries)
6. Alzheimer's disease
7. Diabetes mellitus

(See Hoyert & Xu, 2012, who compiled data for the U.S. Department of Health and Human Services: CDC National Center for Health Statistics.)

The DNR order reflects what a terminally ill patient *does not* want done to prolong life. Many health-care providers believe it gives a negative, crisis-oriented connotation to the patient, family, and members of the interprofessional health-care team. The DNR order implies no further interventions will occur when illness begins to overwhelm bodily functions. However, this assessment becomes murky given that six of the top seven leading causes of death are due to chronic disease.

A proposed revision of the DNR order, the AND describes what *will* occur if resuscitation attempts are needed. This welcome change focuses on alleviating suffering and providing care to comfort a patient. This order reassures patients, families, and members of the health-care team of every effort to keep patients comfortable, promote palliation, and provide for early discussion of EOL choices rather than crisis interventions during an arrest. This type of order assists in providing EOL care to patients with long-term chronic illness in which a steady decline, punctuated by exacerbations, often ensues.

Venneman et al. (2008) tested a hypothesis related to "DNR versus AND" with staff nurses, nursing students, and family members with no health-care background. Simply changing the title of the medical order from DNR to AND increased the probability of endorsement by all participants regardless of health-care experience. This finding suggests a more positive influence of family members through their increased confidence in the AND order, along with a resultant decrease in tension and conflict during the consent process. With the shift from physician-focused decision making to collaboration and patient-centered care, the concept of the AND order can include all stakeholders.

In 2004, Matzo, an EOL care expert, described the process of death and dying as "peri-death." Similar to the process of a surgical intervention (preoperative, intraoperative, and postoperative phases = perioperative period), the peri-death period encompasses the process of biological changes, signs and symptoms, beliefs, or responses at any step in the process of dying. Peri-death may last days, months, or years and includes a prolonged decline in health, a steady decline secondary to an acute terminal illness, or a sudden death.

The death phase includes pronouncement of a patient's death, postmortem care, organ procurement, and care of survivors. It is important to consider physical, psychosocial, cultural, and spiritual needs of patients and survivors. After a patient's death, the care of survivors continues according to the agency involved in EOL care and may last from minutes to years.

The first phase of peri-death is the diagnosis of:
- An acute, terminal illness (e.g., pancreatic cancer).
- Exacerbation and end-stage events of a chronic illness (e.g., chronic kidney disease from type 2 diabetes mellitus).
- Sudden death of a patient from an injury or acute illness (e.g., motor vehicle accident or bacterial meningitis).

This initial phase occurs when death is inevitable and life-preserving measures are withdrawn. Interventions to provide comfort and alleviate fear become the most important nursing actions. Patients have reported their fear of dying comes from concerns about lack of pain control, dyspnea, and emotional distress from burdening their family or dying alone.

Nurses address these concerns through patient advocacy, encouraging all members of an interprofessional health-care team to work together to alleviate suffering and allay patients' fears as death approaches.

Actively dying patients show specific signs and symptoms as their physiological processes deteriorate. Peripheral edema, difficulty swallowing, and emotional withdrawal are common. The time it takes for a patient's body systems to shut down can range from 24 hours to 10 to 14 days. Table 8–5, "Body System Failure on Imminent Death," provides an explanation of this deterioration for each body system.

As a patient nears death, the nurse and the family members can watch for predictable signs and symptoms of impending death:

- Change in the patient's level of consciousness.
- Collection of fluids in the mouth and throat ("death rattle").
- Respirations with mandibular movement.
- Cyanosis to the extremities.
- Inability to palpate the radial pulse.

Before these signs occur, ask your patients and family members if they would like to share stories of the past, discuss burial wishes or organ donation (see Table 8–6, "Organ Donation and Procurement"), or say good-bye. When death is imminent, it becomes more difficult for patients to communicate and for the nurse or family members to understand patients' faltering speech. Additionally, seek to understand the wishes of family members near the time of death. This proactive approach educates family members about the nurse's role as patient advocate and allows

Table 8–5 Body System Failure on Imminent Death

BODY SYSTEM	SIGNS AND SYMPTOMS	PATHOPHYSIOLOGY
Cardiovascular	Decreased blood volume; quiet Korotkoff sounds Early: Tachycardia Late: Bradycardia and low BP Decrease in peripheral circulation; clammy; becomes mottled in appearance over soles of feet and bony prominences (late) Cool skin; normal core temperature Delirium Edema, nausea, pain	Dehydration; difficulty swallowing fluids Hypoxia; dehydration; decreased blood volume Slowing metabolism Dehydration Third-spacing of fluids

Table 8–5 Body System Failure on Imminent Death—cont'd

BODY SYSTEM	SIGNS AND SYMPTOMS	PATHOPHYSIOLOGY
Respiratory	Diminished or adventitious breath sounds; "death rattle" (late) Air hunger and restlessness (dyspnea) Irregular and shallow respirations alternating with apnea	Impaired cardiac function; lymphatic and pulmonary congestion with decreased protein levels in the blood Increased levels of CO_2
Musculoskeletal	Weakness, mouth droop, difficulty swallowing; muscles of tongue and soft palate sag; gag and clearing of pharynx decrease (late) producing "death rattle"	Poor nutritional status for effective muscle strength and functioning
Renal	Decreased urinary output Incontinence	Decreased cardiac output Muscles of sphincters relax
Neurological and Other	Fear, pain, social withdrawal Agitation/delirium	Refusing to eat or drink Psychosocial and cultural beliefs Electrolyte or glucose abnormalities, organ failure, drugs, stool impaction, infections, metastases

Table 8–6 Organ Donation and Procurement

QUESTIONS	ANSWERS
What national organizations are involved in organ transplantation?	United Network for Organ Sharing (UNOS); Organ Procurement and Transplantation Network (OPTN)
Who can donate?	Living donors; donation after brain death; donation after cardiac death
What are absolute exclusions to organ donation?	HIV-positive; active cancer; systemic infection
What can be donated?	Whole body, organs, tissue, stem cells, blood

Continued

Table 8–6 Organ Donation and Procurement—cont'd	
QUESTIONS	ANSWERS
When can donation occur?	Living donors; donation after brain death; donation after cardiac death
Where does organ transplantation take place?	Transplant centers throughout the United States
How can patients help?	Patients make family aware of their wishes; chaplains, ethics staff, or nurses discuss option with patients and their families
Why is the need so great?	As of August 1, 2008, 99,252 patients were in need of a transplant; during the first 5 months of 2008, 5,800 people donated an organ

both patients and survivors to experience death as close to their expectations as possible.

Nurses typically witness death more frequently than most individuals. Family members who have never lost a loved one may be inconsolable or have unexpected actions, such as shaking a patient to "wake him up," hitting another family member for explaining their loved one has died, or climbing into the hospital bed to hold the patient. At the time of death, it is important for the nurse to express sympathy to family members by saying, "I am sorry for your loss." Ask survivors if they would like some time with the deceased. Allow time for them to grieve together in the presence of their loved one, which may be the last time for survivors to see and touch the deceased.

After final goodbyes, postmortem care begins. This phase includes bathing the patient, organ procurement, and other actions according to hospital or agency policy and procedure. A short debriefing for survivors, including examination of the nurse's own reactions, can help ease the psychological and spiritual stress encountered while caring for a dying loved one or patient. This step rarely happens but could provide great comfort and care for caregivers, many of whom have extended themselves during their loved one's terminal illness.

ALERT

Recognize and report suicide ideation, psychological breakdown, and other emergencies where patients are at risk to do harm to themselves or others.

PEAK PERFORMANCE: GRIEF

Nurses have a profound opportunity to apply their pattern recognition for grief and their natural inclination for empathy to improve outcomes for grieving patients and families. Increase your overall understanding of grief with our PEAK mnemonic to summarize nursing process, use best evidence, and promote the following desired outcomes:

- A full, safe, and authentic exploration of grief when indicated with recipients of care.
- Provision of empathy in addition to problem solving.
- Prevention of the sequelae arising from prolonged grief.

P—Purpose

- Counter providers' tendencies to ignore, dismiss, elicit information, or problem solve when recipients of care express strong emotion such as grief.
- Support identification of the negative emotions of grief. Nurses and other providers often address the problem underlying the emotion, especially when the problem involves logistical or biomedical issues, as opposed to the grief itself.

E—Evidence

- Studies have repeatedly found that providers miss 70% to 90% of opportunities to express empathy.
- Patients report "missed nursing care" includes failing to listen to them.

A—Action

- Assist recipients of care to express positive and negative emotions related to grief-producing events.
- Identify explicit indications of emotion, such as whenever patients name the emotion itself.
- Recognize implicit indications of emotion, such as whenever patients discuss an emotional situation, including death or illness of a loved one, significant life concerns or changes (e.g., lost job, unable to pay bills), or diagnoses of serious illness (e.g., cancer).
- Offer patients bereavement guidance, such as (a) setting a timer to grieve openly and authentically for 30 minutes on day 1, for 29 minutes on day 2, for 28 minutes on day 3, and so on, and (b) seeking further professional help when grief interferes with activities of daily living after a month or other context-dependent time frame.

K—Knowledge

Emotions of grief are context dependent and highly individualized. Emotions that interfere with a return to activities of daily living include:

- Anguish—the experience of excruciating distress, suffering, or pain, which becomes unbearable and may provoke pathophysiological responses and reactions.

Continued

PEAK PERFORMANCE: GRIEF—cont'd

- Pining—the experience of suffering with longing, which creates a denial of reality.
- Prolonged anger or rage—an initially energizing feeling, which now provokes exhaustion or inappropriate behavior.
- The emotion underlying prolonged anger or rage—feeling betrayed by one's choices, lifestyle, body, or the health-care system, which are now beyond a grieving person's control.

CLINICAL VOICE: THE IMPORTANCE OF NURSING PRESENCE IN END-OF-LIFE CARE

While I was completing my senior practicum, I realized that my preceptor had something to offer patients that I wasn't going to learn in a book and maybe not in my first few years as a nurse. She had a calm way of sitting down with each patient and family just to talk. I watched and listened while I worked on the many tasks that crammed the mental schedule I had set for each patient.

After passing the NCLEX-RN, I pursued a position in the hospital system where I had worked as a CNA, but I also trained to be a hospice volunteer. I realized I needed more than the nursing student's task-oriented busyness to connect with my patients. I knew I needed to develop my own compassionate presence.

I've enjoyed my RN position at the hospital as well as my hospice volunteer work. As a hospice volunteer, I visit "my" assigned hospice patient weekly, providing compassionate presence, advocacy, and respite for families. I've also had the honor of taking shifts to stay with patients who are actively dying, either to provide respite for the family, caregivers, and chaplains or simply to make sure a person without family and friends does not die alone.

When I visit patients and family I am fulfilling that original goal of developing my nursing presence, but hospice has become so much more for me. I've connected with the beautiful souls of my patients, learned a lot about myself, made friends with other volunteers, and felt included as part of the interdisciplinary care team that wraps each hospice patient (and family) in support and understanding. Patients use palliative care and hospice services to make the last part of their life as happy and pain-free as possible, some for a week or two and many for 6 months or longer.

My hospice work has helped me become a better hospital nurse and patient advocate, as I see the continuum of nursing care and guidance. Just as many terminally ill patients have to change long-held hopes and plans, many patients want to make a transition from hospital care to hospice care. Nurses, case managers, and physicians can ease these difficult decisions and discussions, if we are willing to sit down and be present for just a minute . . . Mary Fiore, BSN, RN

Chapter Summary

This chapter focused on the response of nurses to critical patient situations, including changing patient conditions, pain management, and end-of-life care. In the next chapter, we present issues of health-care ethics, including principles, real-life experiences, and emerging areas affecting the nursing profession. Those areas include genomics, go-green initiatives, nanotechnologies (electronic devices), and more stringent rules and regulations governing health-care delivery, such as the Health Insurance Portability and Accountability Act (HIPAA).

9 Ethics: Addressing Dilemmas in Professional Practice

CHAPTER 9

Ethics: Addressing Dilemmas in Professional Practice

To fulfill the promise of the art and science of professional nursing, an ethical framework is required. This chapter acknowledges the value of comprehensive ethical codes and emphasizes the themes of professional pride, competence, and reflective practice. Finally, it presents two content areas that have major relevance for professional nursing: genomics and "green" (ecological) initiatives.

Ethical Principles

Comprehensive ethical codes derive from ethical principles. Although some principles receive more or less emphasis in nursing programs, the following principles are important in health-care delivery:

- **Beneficence (and nonmaleficence):** Do good, and avoid evil.
- **Common good:** Respect persons, social welfare, and peace and security.
- **Distributive justice:** Grant equitable access to the basic health care necessary for living a fully human life.
- **Human dignity:** Honor the intrinsic worth of every human being, which is the basis for human rights.
- **Informed consent:** Provide the right and responsibility of every competent individual to advance his or her own welfare, exercised freely and voluntarily by consenting or refusing consent to recommended medical procedures, based on a sufficient knowledge of the benefits, burdens, and risks involved.

- **Integrity and totality:** Consider the well-being of the whole person in decisions about any therapeutic intervention or use of technology.
- **Proportionate and disproportionate means:** Fulfill the obligation to preserve life by making use of ordinary means without obligation for use of extraordinary means.
- **Religious or spiritual freedom:** Grant competent individuals the right to act in a manner consistent with their religious or spiritual beliefs.
- **Respect for autonomy:** Acknowledge individuals' capacity for self-determination and their right to make choices and take action based on their values and belief system.
- **Respect for persons:** Treat individuals as free and responsible persons in proportion to their ability in the circumstances at hand.
- **Stewardship:** Appreciate the Earth, with all its natural resources, and human nature, with its biopsychosocial and spiritual capacities.

Ethical principles do not exist in isolation. In the following feature, one situation is described where competing principles required advocacy, scrutiny, application, and honor.

💬 CLINICAL VOICE: WHEN ETHICAL PRINCIPLES CLASH

Mrs. Edgar, a 47-year-old wife, mother, and teacher, was a patient in the intensive care unit because of significant blood loss from a surgical procedure. She had declared her religious affiliation as a Jehovah's Witness and refused blood transfusions. She stated she would rather die. Two days later, she required mechanical ventilation to support her oxygen needs and could not speak. She was able to answer yes and no and write short messages. She continued to affirm that she would rather die than receive blood transfusions.

Nurse Garth knew that Mrs. Edgar's condition was critical. She also believed Mrs. Edgar was competent and entitled to consideration for two ethical principles in particular: religious freedom and respect for autonomy. Nurse Garth decided to call the hospital's ethics board for support. Her advocacy resulted in a meeting of Mr. Edgar, church elders, physicians, the nurse manager, and board representatives. The conversation centered on a clash between two ethical principles: the principle of proportionate and disproportionate means and the principle of religious freedom. Mrs. Edgar's surgeon saw blood transfusion as proportionate, and Mr. Edgar and the church elders presented their faith-based directive against receiving blood and reiterated Mrs. Edgar's wishes.

The surgeon presented the risks related to not receiving blood and described alternative measures already in place to keep Mrs. Edgar from going

> ### 🗨 CLINICAL VOICE: WHEN ETHICAL PRINCIPLES CLASH—cont'd
>
> into hemorrhagic shock, including rapid infusion of IV fluids. He requested insertion of an arterial line to monitor her blood pressure and facilitate laboratory draws.
>
> When Mr. Edgar and the church elders saw blood in the arterial line during a draw for arterial blood gas interpretation, they questioned the nurse. Nurse Garth stated her sensitivity to Mrs. Edgar's religious beliefs and said she had called for their meeting with the ethics board. Then she described the purpose of the blood draw, explained that Mrs. Edgar would not receive anyone else's blood from this line, and demonstrated the flush technique, which would keep the line patent and not allow blood that had exited her body to return. Satisfied that his wife's care respected their religious beliefs, Mr. Edgar went home to sleep for the first time since his wife's surgery.
>
> Mrs. Edgar recovered slowly and without further complications. Three weeks later Nurse Garth received a letter of appreciation from the Edgars. The next year, Nurse Garth learned of a "bloodless" surgery program that would intentionally minimize the need for blood transfusions. She successfully applied to become the program's clinical nurse educator and sensitized many more nurses to advocate for their patients' religious beliefs.

Code of Ethics for Nurses

Ethical codes facilitate thorough evaluation of dilemmas that present with enough lead time to consider multiple approaches and optimal outcomes. Nursing education in the United States steeps students in the nine provisions of the American Nurses Association *Code of Ethics*, published in 2001 after a 6-year process of review, analysis, and revision of its 1985 *Code for Nurses*. Detailed directives and interpretative statements accompany the provisions, making them foundational to the process of becoming a registered nurse. Other countries, including Canada and Australia, and several professional nursing organizations also have codes. In our view, however, these lengthy codes are too cumbersome for addressing dilemmas that occur in everyday practice. Nurses need concise guidance to make day-to-day ethical decisions.

The International Council of Nurses (ICN) offers such concise guidance in its *Code of Ethics for Nurses, revised* (2012). With just four elements, the ICN code is readily committed to memory and provides an accessible framework for reflective practice. Each element connects nurses to a broader focus:

- **Nurses and people:** The nurse has primary professional responsibility to people requiring nursing care.

- **Nurses and practice:** The nurse carries personal responsibility and accountability for nursing practice and for maintaining competence through lifelong learning.
- **Nurses and the profession:** The nurse assumes the major role in determining and implementing acceptable standards of clinical nursing practice, management, research, and education.
- **Nurses and coworkers:** The nurse sustains a cooperative relationship with coworkers in nursing and other fields.

The fourth point contains an explicit statement of advocacy for recipients of care: "The nurse takes appropriate action to safeguard individuals, families, and communities when their health is endangered by a coworker or any other person." "Coworker" includes other nurses; nurses value the notion of connection to one another through a commonly held, international ethical code. The box below lists the principles of this ethical code.

EVIDENCE FOR PRACTICE: PRINCIPLES IN ICN CODE

The need for nursing is universal.

Nurses promote health, prevent illness, restore health, and alleviate suffering.

Inherent in nursing is respect for human rights.

Nurses render health services to the individual, the family, and the community.

Nurses coordinate their services with those of related groups.

Ethical Considerations in Professional Nursing

Research about ethical dilemmas in nursing emerged in the 1980s and focused on nurses' personal dilemmas and moral reasoning. In the 1990s, research explored broader themes for the nursing profession. A study in 1991 elicited the five most frequent ethical issues:

- Inadequate staffing patterns.
- Prolonged life with heroic measures.
- Inappropriate resource allocation.
- Inappropriate discussion of patient cases.
- Colleagues' irresponsible activity.

These ethical issues persist in the explosion of expectations for nurses' expertise in numerous content areas. Whether referred to as competencies, hallmarks of excellence, or indicators, these areas feature nurse-sensitive elements that require ethical decision making in daily practice. These content areas come from the American Association of Colleges of Nursing, National League for Nursing, Joint Commission, Institute of Medicine, and QSEN Institute:

- Geriatrics/gerontology.
- Genomics.
- Global awareness.
- End-of-life care.
- Evidence-based practice.
- Cultural humility and human diversity.
- Informatics, health-care technologies, and nanotechnologies.
- Emergency preparedness.
- Patient safety.
- Safe handling of patients.
- Patient-centered care.
- Interprofessional teamwork and collaboration.
- Quality improvement.
- Ecological/green initiatives.
- Community-based practice.
- Dimensional analysis for drug calculations.
- High-fidelity simulation.

Nurse educators, in the process of developing curricula related to these competencies, must ensure these educational strategies are evidence-based and accessible to students with disabilities. Thanks to advances in assistive technologies, such as enhanced stethoscopes, students with visual and hearing impairments have been able to soar as nurses. Often, they bring an extra measure of determination and compassion to the profession, and they serve as role models to young patients striving to find capabilities within, or despite, disabilities.

Of these content areas, we have selected two for further exploration in this chapter because of their relative newness and explicit connection to ethical practice: genomics and ecological/green initiatives. (See Chapter 1 for a discussion of evidence-based practice, patient safety, and quality improvement; see Chapter 2 for a presentation of dimensional analysis for drug calculations; and see Chapter 7 for a discussion of interprofessional teamwork, collaboration, and I-SBAR-R.)

Genomics

Genomics (pronounced juh-NO-mix) was defined by scientists in 1987 as the study of the function and interaction of all the genes in the human genome. In 2003, scientists completed the Human Genome Map. By 2006, they had described 16,127 autosomal conditions and offered 1,317 genetic tests. Genomic medicine ranges from a prenatal focus on a single gene mutation to an adult focus on multifactorial lifestyle diseases such as diabetes and heart disease.

The ability of nurses to understand genomics and related ethical implications comes from many sources. Chief among them are:

- Jean F. Jenkins, PhD, RN, FAAN, of the National Human Genome Research Institute of the National Institutes of Health, a nurse and Fellow in the American Academy of Nursing (FAAN), nursing's highest honor.
- The Mayo Clinic, which holds national conferences that feature nurses working directly in genomics (www.mayoclinic.com).
- Sigma Theta Tau's *Journal of Nursing Scholarship,* which fulfilled a 2-year commitment to "genomics for health," beginning in the second quarter of 2005 (Volume 37, Issue Number 2), and which continues to publish related evidence-based literature. For example, in 2013, this journal published articles (Volume 45, Issue Number 1) about genomics and:
  - Cancer care.
  - Metabolic syndrome.
  - Cardiovascular topics (myocardial infarction and coronary artery disease, stroke, and sudden cardiac death).
  - Autism spectrum disorder.
  - Current and emerging technology approaches.
  - Adults with neuropsychiatric conditions.
  - Ethical, legal, and social issues.
- Cincinnati Children's Hospital Medical Center, which houses the Web-based Genetics Education Program for Nurses, helping more than 2,500 nurses to acquire genetic and genomic nursing competencies (http://www.cincinnatichildrens.org/education/clinical/nursing/genetics/default/).
- National Human Genome Research Institute (www.genome.gov), which houses Web-based resources for health professionals, including videos on its "GenomeTV" and numerous articles related to patient care and ethics.

Many students learned terms related to genetics that are necessary but insufficient for an expanded knowledge of genomics. The margin box defines these original terms.

A glossary of terms related to genomics follows. These terms were invented and end in *-ome* because *chromosome* was strongly associated with all things genetic.

EVIDENCE FOR PRACTICE: FAMILIAR TERMS FROM GENETICS

Genes: The units of heredity.

Genetics: The science of human biological variation as it relates to health and disease; the study of the etiology, pathogenesis, and natural history of diseases and disorders that are genetic in origin (e.g., the *BRCA-1* gene is a tumor suppressor gene; associated diseases, owing to a mutation turning off this gene, are breast cancer and ovarian cancer).

Chromosomes: Separate molecules ranging from 50 to 250 million base pairs that contain the genes of a particular organism.

Genomics
- All the genetic material in the chromosomes of a particular organism; all the interaction between genes and between genes and the environment.
- Genomics also describes size of the genome, comparison between sequences, and comparison of gene arrangement on a chromosome between species.
- The human genome contains 3 billion nucleotide bases.

Transcriptome and transcriptomics
- **Transcriptome:** The RNA expressed by a cell or organ at a particular time in particular conditions (RNA molecules).
- **Transcriptomics:** The study of the full set of RNA encoded by the genome.

Proteome and proteomics
- **Proteome:** The proteins expressed by a cell or organ at a particular time in specific conditions.
- **Proteomics:** The study of the full set of proteins encoded by a genome (e.g., tissue banks are studying proteins of liver cancer, mapping them, and trying to find out what goes wrong).

Metabalome

- **Metabalome:** The study of metabolites active in a cell, organ, or organism at a particular time in specific conditions.

Genomics has astonishing implications for health care, especially in the areas of individualized treatments, mutations, pharmacotherapeutics, and molecular diagnostics. Genetic testing can diagnose a disease, confirm a clinical diagnosis, provide prognostic information about the course of the disease, diagnose asymptomatic individuals, and predict risk of disease in progeny. The emerging field of pharmacogenomics, which will revolutionize information in drug handbooks, concerns the ability to correlate DNA variation with response to pharmacological treatment. Benefits will include avoidance of adverse drug reactions, avoidance of drugs that are not efficacious, and choice of drugs that are efficacious. Gene therapy offers the potential of using genes to treat disease or enhance particular traits.

Genomics has dramatically altered understanding of mutations and their implications. Classes of mutations include the following:

- Point mutations (e.g., hereditary hemochromatosis [HHEMO] has few mutations, whereas cystic fibrosis transmembrane regulation [CFTR] has more than 1,300 mutations throughout the gene, such as changes in conformation, which can be a bubble, bend, or bulge).
- Large deletions, duplications, or insertions (e.g., α-thalassemia).
- Trinucleotide repeat expansions (e.g., fragile X).
- Imprinting/methylation (e.g., Prader-Willi/Angelman syndrome).

Diagnostic tools for mutations include probes, fluorescence resonance energy transfer (FRET), melt-curves, array technologies, mutation scanning techniques, DNA sequencing, assays, methylation, and electrophoresis. The Mayo Clinic continues its leadership in the field of genomics through its extraordinary Center for Individualized Medicine. More recent diagnostic advances include:

- The discovery of molecular markers, called biomarkers, in blood and tissue, which aid in more precise disease diagnosis and treatment.
- Clinomics, which moves discoveries from the laboratory to patient care using practical, cost-effective genomic tests.

In the future, technology for personalized medicine will include high-throughput DNA sequencing and analytes, such as DNA methylation profiling and microRNAs.

Nurses have already become more involved in ordering genetic tests and interpreting test results. Reasons for referral are receiving new scrutiny for a genetic basis or component. See the Clinical Voice for a likely scenario and ethical implications.

CLINICAL VOICE: ETHICAL CONSIDERATIONS

At his yearly physical examination, Mr. Green, 62 years old, had abnormal liver enzyme function test results. His hepatitis screen was negative. A second-tier screen revealed elevated serum ferritin: 2,000 ng/mL (normal range, 22 to 3?? ng/mL).

Question: Is the elevated iron in this patient due to a defect in the *HFE* gene?

Referral: Evaluation of hereditary hemochromatosis (autosomal recessive disorder, which requires a mutation in both paired genes).

Method: Polymerase chain reaction (PCR)–based assay.

Result: C282Y homozygous (two copies of the C282Y mutation identified).

Interpretation: Diagnosis confirmed.

Management: Phlebotomy with annual serum transferrin saturation and serum ferritin levels.

Patient education: Comprehensive assessment followed by lay-language explanations of condition and treatment.

Ethical considerations: Sensitive discussion with Mr. Green, who did not want to "burden" his two adult daughters with his diagnosis. The nurse drew on Mr. Green's empathetic nature by using lay terms to explain "respect for autonomy." This ethical principle advocates giving people information and allowing them to make their own decisions. Mr. Green weighed his desire to remain a "strong and healthy father figure" against the 25% risk of recurrence in his children. He assessed the risk as significant and decided to tell his daughters. The nurse offered him sample wording: "Daughter, you have a 1 in 4 chance of having the malfunctioning genes and developing this disease. You have a 1 in 2 chance of having one abnormal gene, which would make you a carrier." Mr. Green later reported that both daughters opted for genetic testing, which showed neither one had inherited the abnormal gene. He also said he had become closer to them. They did look at him in a new light, not as sick or needy but as mortal and unselfish. His daughters took turns driving him to his phlebotomy appointments, and he cherished this time with them.

The Clinical Voice suggests the scope of challenges for nurses in the field of genomics. Nurses must inform themselves about genomics (see Box 9–1, "Appreciating Human Complexity"); keep pace with rapid changes in the field; and learn new approaches in patient education, such as lay-language analogies and metaphors, therapeutic communication strategies about inherited conditions, and empathetic ways to share sensitive information with family members. Attending to the

---

Box 9–1 Appreciating Human Complexity

- The average gene consists of 3,000 bases (the largest gene, dystrophin, has 2.4 million bases).
- There are 20,000 to 30,000 human genes (a recent guess from Sweden is 23,700 human genes).
- Functions of about 50% of the genes are unknown. For example, 10 genes are needed to activate vitamin B_{12}.
- The human genome is 99.9% the same in all human beings. The human genome is 99.5% the same for Cro-Magnon as for Neanderthal. One change in a gene can have dramatic phenotypic expression.
- About 2% of the genome encodes instructions for protein synthesis.
- Genes are concentrated in a random area along the genome, separated by what scientists refer to as "junk," which may mean "not understood."
- According to the National Library of Medicine, Chromosome 1 (the largest) likely contains 2,000 to 2,100 genes that provide instructions for making proteins. Chromosome Y (the smallest, but which has many functions) likely contains 50 to 60 genes that provide instructions for making proteins.
- Repeat sequences that do not code for protein comprise about 50% of the human genome. Scientists believe repeat sequences have no direct functions but shed light on chromosome structure and dynamics. Over time, these repeat sequences reshape the genome by rearranging it, creating new genes, and reshuffling old genes.

---

following recommendations will accelerate your mastery in this emerging area:

- Review the genomics competencies for nursing practice by the American Nurses' Association (ANA), which are available at the ANA Web site (www.nursingworld.org) or at the Web site of the International Society of Nurses in Genetics (www.isong.org).
- Learn terms—patterns (autosomal-dominant, autosomal-recessive, x-linked); new or de novo mutations; atypical inheritance (mitochondrial inheritance, imprinting, uniparental disomy, expanding trinucleotide repeats).
- Collaborate with genetic counselors (nurses' expanded role in patients' response to genetic information).
- Assess family and medication histories, physical findings, environmental factors, and patients' related knowledge and questions.

- Rethink the importance of family history and support the U.S. Surgeon General Family Health History Initiative (http://www.hhs.gov/familyhistory/):
  - Add a pedigree and genogram to the family history.
  - Determine the significance of second-degree and third-degree relatives.
  - Assess for red flags using the mnemonic *GENES*: *G* = group of congenital anomalies; *E* = extreme or exceptional presentation of common conditions; *N* = neurodevelopmental delay or degeneration; *E* = extreme or exceptional pathology; *S* = surprising laboratory values.
- Learn genetic screening tools: See the related Coach Consult: The "SCREEN" Approach.
- Educate patients: A patient had a clean colonoscopy, but DNA evaluation of a stool sample showed cancer cells from the esophagus. The patient understandably thought the colonoscopy had gone all the way to the esophagus.

The use of genomic discoveries in reproductive testing and genetic enhancement lacks consensus. Nurses can increase their value as stakeholders through considering the four elements of the ICN *Code of Ethics for Nurses*, shown earlier in this chapter, and reviewing related federal policy (www.genome.gov):

- **Genetic discrimination.** Most states have laws to protect the public from genetic discrimination by insurance companies and laws to protect their citizens from genetic discrimination in the workplace. According to the federal Genetic Discrimination Fact Sheet, "Genetic discrimination occurs if people are treated unfairly because of differences in their DNA that increase their chances of getting a certain disease. For example, a health insurer might refuse to give coverage to a woman who has a DNA difference that raises her odds of getting breast cancer. Employers also could use DNA information to decide whether to hire or fire workers."
- **National action.** 1990—Americans With Disabilities Act passes and provides protection from discrimination for "genetically disabled" people;

ALERT

Follow Health Insurance Portability and Accountability Act (HIPAA) rules: Keep relatives' names out of permanent medical records, and obtain relatives' permission and consent according to the presenting situation.

275

1996—HIPAA provides some protection from discrimination but does not go far enough related to genetic information; 2000—an executive order prohibits genetic discrimination in the workplace for federal employees; 2003—U.S. Senate passes the Genetic Information Nondiscrimination Act, which protects Americans against discrimination based on their genetic information when it comes to health insurance and employment, but it does not become law; 2005—a similar Senate bill, Genetic Information Non-Discrimination Act, passes but stalls in House committees; 2008—Genetic Information Nondiscrimination Act (GINA) passes after Congressional debate spanning 13 years and paves the way for people to take full advantage of the promise of personalized medicine without fear of discrimination; 2010—The Affordable Care Act establishes a "guaranteed issue," whereby issuers offering insurance in either the group or individual market must provide coverage for all individuals who request it and prohibits issuers from discriminating against patients with genetic diseases by refusing coverage because of "pre-existing conditions."

- **Questions confronting lawmakers and insurance companies.** If no symptoms exist, why should insurance companies pay for genetic newborn screening? If genetics begins at conception, what are the impact and explanation of "pre-existing condition," especially when predisposition does not equal disease?

Genomics soon will affect every setting of health-care delivery. Your engagement in this topic can be accidental or intentional. The latter choice will not only accelerate your progression to competent nurse but will also set you apart from peers unfamiliar with this emerging focus. The Clinical Voice box, Ethical Considerations, shows how genomics will have implications across health-care settings. Ethical considerations must move from an afterthought to an integral part of the practice of nursing.

💬 CLINICAL VOICE: ETHICAL CONSIDERATIONS

Mr. Brooks, a married father of two adopted children, had inherited cystic fibrosis (CF) from his carrier parents. CF, an autosomal-recessive disease, is relatively common and has an average survival age of about 35 years based on ages of patients in the CF Foundation Patient Registry and the distribution of deaths in 2009. Nurses see patients with CF in pediatric, adolescent, and adult medicine; in ambulatory and inpatient settings; and in intensive care and transplant units.

Mr. Brooks was diagnosed at age 2 years, and subsequent genetic testing revealed he had the R117H mutation on chromosome 7. Now at age 34 years, he had an understanding of the severity of his disease balanced with a profound drive to live his best life. He had seen the power of nursing involved in helping him recover from respiratory infections over the years and readily connected with nurses to promote desired outcomes. Although he endured one to three hospitalizations a year, he counted himself lucky to be among the 15% who did not also experience digestive problems. He was well aware of approaching the average survival age, and recent symptoms and diagnostic tests indicated he had end-stage CF.

As the transplant coordinator at a university hospital, Nurse Jordan was part of the team evaluating Mr. Brooks for a bilateral lung transplant. Through years of experience, the team had identified the need for explicit ethical analysis of each individual case referred for transplant. Principles of distributive justice, informed consent, integrity and totality, proportionate and disproportionate means, and respect for autonomy were central to their transplant evaluations, and a formal ethics board reviewed actual and potential clashes related to physical, financial, and emotional burdens for patients and their families.

Mr. Brooks was accepted and eventually received a bilateral lung transplant without medical complications. As he and the team addressed ethical implications in advance, he also managed potential burdens as anticipated. Although his medication regimen was daunting, Mr. Brooks returned to his family, employment, and hobbies with a much improved quality of life.

Ecological/Green Initiatives

The second content area of discussion in this chapter is ecological/green initiatives. As with genomics, this burgeoning focus for nursing has broad ethical implications.

Stewardship has emerged as a synthesis principle of ethics because of its dual emphasis on the Earth, with all its natural resources, and human nature, with its biological, psychological, social, and spiritual capacities. Nurses in every setting, from home health to the operating room, have an opportunity to exercise stewardship, particularly to capture the momentum of "go-green" initiatives. Nurses can have a profound impact in their settings to reduce waste, conserve resources, and promote sustainability in health-care delivery and beyond. The box below describes one recent effort. In addition, the Luminary Project (http://www.theluminaryproject.org/) identifies nurses around the United States who have advanced the causes of green nursing. Dr. Gary Laustsen, a co-author of this textbook, has one such Web site (available from: http://www.theluminaryproject.org/story.php?detail = 95).

Concern for environmental protection has recurred throughout history. For example, in the Middle East, the earliest known writings about the environment addressed contamination of air, soil, and water. In the early 13th century, King Edward I of England proclaimed a ban on the burning of sea-coal in London because of pollution from its smoke. In the United States, environmental activism has its roots in the thought of the 1830s and 1840s, made famous through the writings of Henry David Thoreau. The era of American pragmatism in the latter half of the 19th century expanded attention to the environment through efforts to preserve wilderness areas. National endeavors arose during the Industrial Revolution and catapulted in the 1950s with the recognition of smog. Rachel Carson's compelling book, *Silent Spring*, accelerated momentum in the protection of the environment during the 1970s.

EVIDENCE FOR PRACTICE: PROMOTING ECOLOGICAL BEHAVIOR

Holistic nursing practice provides theoretical and ethical foundations for nursing to prosper and promote a profession learning to "think globally and care locally." One groundbreaking study, conducted in 2004, sought to promote ecological behavior in nurses through Community Based Action Research (CBAR). A convenient, purposive community of 10 nurses at a western, urban hospital, self-identified as "The Green Team," enacted the CBAR design. The research project selected was red bag waste minimization. Actions for the research project were identified, prioritized, evaluated, and revised. Data generated consisted of three types: contextual, experiential, and action-related. Data were organized into three categories: research process, participants, and project.

A team approach promoted and achieved improved changes to ecologically related nursing practices. The team developed an informed awareness of the implications of nurse-generated waste through active waste analysis. The team promoted a change in the hospital's infectious waste policy. Barriers required a revision of goals and redirected research activities.

Findings suggested that an ecological view be incorporated into nursing education. Promoting nurses' ecological behavior through action research was realized.

Since the mid-1970s, the U.S. Resource Conservation and Recovery Act (RCRA) has been the primary law governing the disposal of solid and hazardous waste. Congress passed RCRA on October 21, 1976, to address the increasing problems the nation faced from growing volumes of municipal and industrial waste. RCRA, which amended the Solid Waste Disposal Act of 1965, gives the U.S. Environmental Protection Agency the authority to control hazardous waste and set national goals for:

- Protecting human health and the environment from the potential hazards of waste disposal.
- Conserving energy and natural resources.
- Reducing the amount of waste generated.
- Ensuring the management of waste in an environmentally sound manner.

Readiness for "go-green" initiatives emerged in nursing in the early 1990s. Hospitals for a Healthy Environment (H2E) began as a collaborative effort among the Environmental Protection Agency, American Hospital Association, ANA, and Health Care Without Harm. In 2008, this effort was reorganized and renamed *Practice Greenhealth* to reflect its new role as a membership organization that promotes environmentally sustainable practices and prevention of pollution in health-care facilities. An organization with membership open to individual nurses is the Alliance of Nurses for Healthy Environments (http://envirn.org/). For example, nurses throughout the United States have initiated innovative programs to:

- Reduce the use of equipment containing the toxic chemical DEPH in neonatal intensive care units.
- Repackage hospital supplies in an environmentally conscious manner.
- Recycle mercury-filled batteries.

Another national membership organization is the National Recycling Coalition (NRC). This nonprofit organization represents and advocates for every sector of the recycling industry in the United States. In 2002, the NRC added a fourth "R" to the motto, "Reduce-Reuse-Recycle," which receives prominent coverage on the Web site of the U.S. Environmental Protection Agency. The fourth "R" stands for "Rethink." Project C.U.R.E. (Commission on Urgent Relief and Equipment) embodies one of the most outstanding efforts to "rethink" medical surplus and waste.

Project C.U.R.E. (www.projectcure.org) identifies, solicits, sorts, and distributes medical supplies and services according to the needs of the world. In true nursing process fashion, Project C.U.R.E. completes an on-site assessment in countries requesting aid and establishes partnerships with governmental agencies to prevent corruption and graft, including black market redistribution of delivered supplies. Since the first shipment to Brazil in 1987, Project C.U.R.E. has shipped cargo containers to more than 120 countries, and all shipments have reached their intended recipients.

Project C.U.R.E. has redistributed items ranging from bath basins to sterile gloves to entire heart catheterization laboratories. The need is urgent in all developing countries. For example:

- In Kenya, an area of growing HIV/AIDS infection, nurses boil used needles over a fire before reusing them.
- In Nepal, a premature newborn lies in a worn-out incubator. The machine can barely keep the baby warm.
- In Sudan, physicians lack scalpels and blades. They have resorted to using the lids of tin cans to perform surgical procedures. There is no anesthesia.

Yet, in the United States, patterns of waste are astonishing. For example, a hospital ordered 300 logo-embroidered maroon scrub sets for its nurses, in part to promote brand identification in a competitive hospital marketplace. The hospital rejected the scrub sets when the color did not match the desired branding. The manufacturer notified Project C.U.R.E. of the rejected scrub sets. Instead of ending up in a landfill, the sets were distributed by Project C.U.R.E. to a hospital in southern Africa. Nurses there are proud to wear them, despite sporting the embroidered logo of a hospital in the western United States.

Nurses can make a significant contribution to Project C.U.R.E. as volunteers in its collection and sorting centers, which are located throughout the United States. Nurses recognize donated supplies and correctly sort them for repackaging according to assessed needs throughout the developing world. Nurses everywhere can obtain Project C.U.R.E. collection containers for their units.

The newest trend is to upcycle. Whereas recycling makes the same product such as aluminum cans over and over, upcycling increases the value of the original product. In simplest terms, upcycling is the practice of taking something that is disposable and transforming it into something of greater use and value:

- Instead of recycling newspaper, wad it up, and place it into work and sport shoes to absorb odors.
- Instead of discarding cans, decorate them as flower pots or pencil cups.
- Instead of throwing plastic bags away, add twill tape handles to make them reusable or braid them into jump ropes, rugs, and sturdy "go-green" tote bags.
- Instead of discarding worn hosiery, donate it to a sewing circle to be made into stuffed animals and puppets for pediatric units.

As a newer nurse, you may have an edge on veteran nurses, many of whom have limited exposure to green initiatives. Demonstrate your access to and investment in ecological content by organizing unit nurses to:

- Initiate a "go-green" committee and identify ways to reduce-reuse-recycle.
- Host a poster competition to "rethink" waste and conservation on your unit.
- Participate in your local community in a visible way by holding a street fair to introduce upcycling.

Then go one step further. Add your leadership skills to track all of the cutting-edge topics:

- Introduce the concept of a journal club. Digest trends, organizational white papers, and research reviews.
- Gather a couple of like-minded colleagues, and develop an in-service in one of the new content areas. Share the work and the rewards of being lifelong learners.
- Notice where you like to put your effort. Consider if a theme emerges suggesting you ought to head for graduate school and an advanced practice role.

Chapter Summary

This chapter focused on ethical issues in nursing practice and explored two current topics, genomics and ecological/green initiatives, and their ethical implications. The next and final chapter offers a balanced approach to self-care and career development. We explain the push for the Doctor of Nursing Practice (DNP) and emphasize benefits from participation in professional nursing organizations. We conclude with take-home messages that accelerate your transition to practicing RN through nursing excellence and professional pride.

10 Next Steps: Advancing in Your Career

CHAPTER 10

Next Steps: Advancing in Your Career

Our final chapter juxtaposes self-care—featuring the cornerstone principle of energy management—and career development. We emphasize motivation and mentorship and offer creative and cut-to-the-chase methods for both topics. We provide our "proven path" to passing the registered nurse licensing examination. We also discuss the value of participating in professional nursing organizations and include "insider" information about how to become a member of the prestigious *Sigma Theta Tau* International Honor Society of Nursing (if you were not inducted during your undergraduate program).

Additionally, we explain the push for the Doctor of Nursing Practice degree and present the recommendation from the American Association of Colleges of Nursing for doctoral preparation to enter future roles in advanced practice nursing. Those roles currently include certified clinical nurse specialists, certified nurse anesthetists, certified nurse midwives, and certified nurse practitioners.

We conclude with a section on promoting nursing excellence and professional pride through this maxim: *Pursue excellence, not perfection.* Our fondest hope is that you will embrace the charge to become "consciously competent." We encourage you to notice where we have emphasized this concept. Then, take one more step to embrace lifelong learning so you can also see yourself as consciously capable throughout your career in professional nursing.

Caring for Self

Self-care for nurses dates from the theoretical perspectives of Careful Nursing, a system of nursing developed in 19th-century Ireland. This theory predates Florence Nightingale and influenced her notions about our metaparadigm, or overall view of nursing. (See Box 10–1, "Establish Your Domain Definition of Nursing.") Our metaparadigm consists of the foundational concepts of professional nursing, which you can recall with the mnemonic *PHEN*:

- *P*erson
- *H*ealth
- *E*nvironment
- *N*ursing

The theory of Careful Nursing offers a model for contemporary nursing practice that explicitly includes self-care. The theory, which Meehan reinterpreted in 2003 from the original system of careful nursing, has 10 major concepts:

1. Disinterested love
2. Contagious calmness
3. Creation of a restorative environment
4. "Perfect" skill in fostering safety and comfort
5. Nursing interventions
6. Health education
7. Participatory-authoritative management
8. Trustworthy collaboration

Box 10–1 Establish Your Domain Definition of Nursing

We propose that you develop a one-sentence statement about what nursing means to you. Adapt one of the following statements, or create your own:

- Nursing is stewardship of holistic human health and healing.
- Nursing is a professional approach to caring for the whole person, inside and out.
- Nursing promotes health and healing across the life span in any setting.

Whatever statement you adopt, try it out on friends and family. You may create newfound respect, especially among people who questioned your career choice out of mainstream impressions of professional nursing. These misperceptions are largely due to the invisibility or misrepresentation of nurses on television shows and lack of direct interaction with nurses in primary care.

Once you have established your "domain definition" of professional nursing, become consciously competent in your approach to practice. Notice that deliberate articulation of nursing process promotes a system akin to muscle memory. When you ritualize your daily practice, you will notice more readily successful strategies in dealing with disruptions to anticipated patterns.

---

9. Power derived from service
10. Nurses care for themselves

The final four concepts of this theory cluster around a theme of personal leadership, which is critical to self-care. One view of leadership is the ability to focus others on the priority of the moment. Notice when and where you have "rallied the troops" to a cause, whether in your personal life or professional endeavors. To accelerate your mastery, we encourage you to see yourself as an emerging leader in as many arenas of your life as possible. Perhaps you:

- Help friends and family members focus on a goal rather than on the numerous or daunting steps required to reach it.
- Provide the vision for a family goal, such as a vacation.
- Take the lead on admissions to your unit.
- Teach a skill or concept that puzzles others.

Seven Motivators

If you already have explicit leadership skills, enhance them with knowledge of motivators, which have varying importance for individuals. For example, some people have a stronger need for achievement than for power. Motivators play a role especially during instruction, whether of patients or colleagues. Seven key motivators are:

1. *Need for achievement:* People want to succeed. Meet and accept colleagues and patients wherever they are, and help them move forward. Ask: What adaptations are needed?

2. *Need for power:* People want to make decisions and seek a modicum of control in any situation. Offer feasible choices when they exist. Ask: Are there two or more acceptable alternatives?

3. *Need for affiliation:* People are social beings and seek interaction. Ask: Would a judicious amount of social interaction benefit this patient? Would my colleagues be more inclined to add current evidence to policies and procedures if we worked in teams of three instead of expecting nurses to work alone?

4. *Need for autonomy:* People desire a balance between freedom and interdependence and between affiliation and independence. Ask: What input is needed to discern a motivating degree of autonomy?

5. *Need for self-esteem:* People may feel good about themselves, but they still seek praise and recognition. More than other motivators, this one depends on your discernment and ability to deliver

valid feedback. Ask: In this situation, will praise be a motivator or a disruptive roadblock to further communication?

6. *Need for safety and security:* As theorized in Maslow's classic hierarchy of needs, people require safety and security to pursue high productivity, achievement, and satisfaction as well as healing. Ask: Have I recognized and dealt with threats to my patients' safety and security? Have I prevented or addressed the three responses to fear: fight, flight, or freeze?

7. *Need for equity:* People expect fair treatment. Ask: Do I convey to patients, families, and colleagues that I am fair, just, and equal in distributing attention and privileges?

In addition to embracing a broad theoretical perspective for self-care, we offer a cut-to-the-chase method of the "four As":

1. Attitude. Dominate your thoughts with positive or neutral attitudes. Challenge any thoughts behind negative feelings, and make a consciously competent effort to move negativity toward neutrality. Although it may be unrealistic or even undesirable to move negativity to positivity, especially around issues of grief and loss, you do not want negativity to turn to wallowing despair. If you think you have little control over your attitude, consider how quickly it would change if someone you wanted to impress walked into the room.

2. Appearance. Value the instantaneous impression of a clean and polished appearance, especially when accompanied by a smile. Your appearance plays an underestimated role in nursing presence. This powerful connection with recipients of care produces "the melt," which you will recognize as a noticeable relaxation of patients and their family members when you enter the room, especially when continuity of care requires repeated interaction. By your appearance, you can also prevent the "meltdown" that sometimes accompanies high-demand situations.

3. Achievement. Strive for personally meaningful achievement and benignly neglect the "shoulds" others may try to impose on you. For example, you might say, "Thank you for caring enough to contribute your thoughts. I'll add them to the options I'm considering." When others' thoughts are unsolicited, unwarranted, or misguided, your reply can still value the givers, even as you discard their opinions. In addition, authentic achievement often

equates with advocacy for your recipients of care. Achievement commonly leads to the next "A," accolades.

4. Accolades. Accept the thanks and praise of others. As a group, nurses tend to be humble, perhaps secondary to the servant-leadership nature of the profession. Consider, however, that you build visibility for the profession when you gratefully accept the honor others seek to bestow on you. Your acceptance speech might include the words of Sir Isaac Newton: "If I have seen further it is by standing on the shoulders of giants."

We also recommend diligent attention to energy management and development of a personally meaningful framework to guide your journey through nursing and life. We explain more about these notions in the next two sections.

EVIDENCE FOR PRACTICE: CONCEPTS IN THE ART OF NURSING

Nursing programs introduce "textbook concepts" associated with the art of nursing, such as caring, compassion, spirituality, advocacy, and presence. In a qualitative study published in 2008, a nurse scientist discovered the following core values, which lend credence to traditional concepts and provide evidence for a more thorough appreciation of the power and purpose of professional nursing:

Caring
Compassion
Spirituality
Community outreach
Providing comfort
Crisis intervention
Going the extra distance

Energy Management

Responsive self-care also depends on the ability to manage your energy, which equates to full engagement in priorities and maintenance of focus on what is truly important. Nurses typically have additional challenges related to energy management because of patients' pressing needs, rotating shifts, limited services during night and weekend shifts, and competing demands on their time when they also are parents or caregivers for their own parents or other relatives. Nola Pender, a prominent nursing leader in the areas of health promotion and disease prevention, theorized six subsets of health:

1. Spiritual growth
2. Health responsibility
3. Physical activity
4. Nutrition
5. Interpersonal relationships
6. Stress management

Taken together, these six subsets represent our overall concept of energy management. To help you make consciously competent decisions in these realms, review Figure 10–1, which depicts the classic conceptualization of "first things first," developed by the late business leader Stephen Covey and his colleagues. The upper right quadrant represents the ideal and often prevents time wasted in other quadrants; time spent in the upper left quadrant must be limited to prevent exhaustion; the lower left quadrant is borderline because of lack of importance and attention on others' priorities; and the lower right quadrant is unacceptable if it keeps you out of the upper right quadrant:

- Upper right quadrant: *INU = Important, Not Urgent:* For example, providing anticipatory guidance to parents or doing an in-service about the value of a journal club.
- Upper left quadrant: *IU = Important, Urgent:* For example, responding to a resuscitation effort or interpreting an arterial blood gas report for a patient having an exacerbation of chronic obstructive pulmonary disease (COPD).
- Lower left quadrant: *NIU = Not Important, Urgent:* For example, responding to e-mails based on chronological order or accessing the latest Facebook postings.
- Lower right quadrant: *NINU = Not Important, Not Urgent:* For example, watching reruns on television or spending more time on a critic than you would on a friend.

WINDOW ON PURSUITS

IU	INU
NIU	NINU

FIGURE 10–1: Covey's Quadrant Model.

PEAK PERFORMANCE: PASSING THE REGISTERED NURSE LICENSING EXAMINATION

Over the years, we have tracked recommendations and results related to passing the registered nurse licensing examination. We present our proven path to success using the PEAK mnemonic:

P—Purpose
- Pass the registered nurse licensing examination when you take it.
- Celebrate your achievement!

E—Evidence
- In the past 5 years, 100% of our graduates have passed the registered nurse licensing examination when they followed our action steps.
- Examination preparation courses and reviews endorse these steps and provide the questions, answers, rationales, practice tests, and test-taking strategies needed to fulfill many of the action steps.

A—Action
- Do well in your nursing school program! We cannot overstate the importance of turning your desire to become a nurse into daily habits of adequate preparation and careful engagement.
- Complete a companion preparation program to immerse yourself in the depth and breadth of professional nursing. If your nursing school does not require or recommend a particular program, purchase a preparation textbook and follow along course by course.
- Answer a sufficient number of examination-style questions from your preparation program before you sit for the test to increase your confidence and reinforce nursing content. Reading rationales, even when you answer questions correctly, will verify you have understood a question as the item-writer intended:
  - A student: 3,000 questions with rationales
  - B student: 4,000 questions with rationales
  - C student: 5,000 questions with rationales
- Do a structured review program of your choosing (textbook, online, in person, downloaded application, or any other approach that meets your needs) because the licensing examination tests safe, advanced beginner practice rather than your nursing school program.
- Manage your energy leading up to the examination and keep disruptions at arm's length—or reschedule. Unexpected failure can occur when you are distracted by uncontrollable events in your personal life, such as a loved one's serious illness. When test questions seem harder than expected, your mind may wander to the reality that your life is harder than expected. This loss of faith and focus is hard to overcome in the already pressurized setting of your licensing examination.

Continued

K—Knowledge

- Know why you want to pass the registered nurse licensing examination:
  - Spend 15 minutes creating a vision board (on a poster or bulletin board) where you post anything that relates to your motivation: photos with family or peers, copies of recommendation letters and job applications, notes of self-encouragement, and inspirational quotations and other messages. Put at least one sticky note on your bathroom mirror for a double effect because you see the note and yourself as you self-encourage: "I will pass the RN licensing examination when I take it!"
  - Keep the self-talk 100% positive. It can take a long time to get your mind to correct a negative emotion, so use motion to control emotion: walk, dance, or jump! Have a go-to theme song that puts you in a happy frame of mind from the first couple of notes and lyrics. Deep breathe in *and* out to expel respiratory acids and other waste products. Encourage peers with signals, pacts, support groups, preparation games or flash cards, and lots of hugs.
- Know yourself and stick to a doable study plan.
  - Use a consistent study approach, such as 3 to 5 hours a day with weekends off.
  - Envision yourself 1 year into safe, competent practice. Then the licensing examination is just a few "important but not urgent" hours out of 1 day on that path.
- Know everything you can about the examination itself:
  - Review the current test plan (available from: www.ncsbn.org).
  - Be aware the first 30 questions are important for the computer's algorithm, so establish your confidence as you sit down to test by saying, "Bring it on!"
  - If you think the test is harder than expected, you are most likely getting questions right. You cannot possibly know, however, so keep doubt at bay.
  - Practice every type of alternative-format question. In particular, have a strategy for questions that ask you to "check all that apply." Treat each potential answer as a true-false statement. Answer it and move to the next potential answer.
  - Know the minimum and maximum number of questions you may face and assume you will have to answer the maximum. Take frequent breaks to maintain energy and focus.

Personal Framework

Have you ever seen a vaudeville act in which the juggler places poles into brackets on a table and then sets plates spinning on top of the poles? His skill lies in rushing back and forth to keep the plates spinning. Without constant attention and due diligence, the plates wobble and eventually fall, crashing to the floor. Many nurses relate to this metaphor when they consider the reality of their lives.

Instead of running around to spin various plates, we recommend articulating a framework based on three concentric rings. The interior-most ring is your self-designated center, or whatever is the most enduring aspect of your life. Movement outward to the next ring expresses who you are. To maintain connection to your center, author Rhonda Byrne recommends recitation of this affirmation: "I am whole, perfect, loving, strong, powerful, harmonious, and happy." We offer a preamble that honors a higher power or creator: "I am grateful, obedient, and devoted." This consciously competent approach could have any number of variations for the affirmations selected. The important feature is the daily reminder to live purposefully and in accordance with time-honored principles.

The second concentric ring represents the micro-level of your life, which encompasses local action. You can make a difference by investing in just one other person. The effect is synergistic, the impact is exponential, and maturity follows from delayed gratification. Actions at the micro-level exemplify the principle of "sowing and reaping," which has three parts:

1. You reap what you sow.
2. You reap much more than you sow.

ALERT

One hundred percent of our students who followed the action steps in our PEAK Performance Box passed the registered nurse licensing examination when they took it. They did not allow a mindset of "passing on the first try," which would tell their brain there could be a second attempt!

COACH CONSULT

A former Jesuit and investment banker, best-selling author Chris Lowney explains one of the most powerful approaches we have encountered to pursue a consciously capable life. His book, *Heroic Leadership*, inspires readers through four pillars of self-leadership that have guided Jesuits for more than 470 years: self-awareness, ingenuity, love, and heroism. His follow-up book, *Heroic Living*, provides an action plan through three foundational pursuits:

1. Articulating a purpose worth the rest of your life, that is, a reason for

Continued

COACH CONSULT —cont'd

living that is so much bigger than yourself that it transforms you, your relationships, and the world as a result.

2. Making wise career and relationship choices.

3. Making each day matter by mindful attention to your actions and results.

Imagine the impact of making these principles and pursuits the cornerstone of your progression through professional nursing!

3. There is a period of waiting between sowing and reaping.

The accompanying Clinical Voice describes one person's effort in developing a guiding framework.

The outermost concentric ring creates the macro-level, where you think globally and with cultural humility about the sustainability of the planet's environmental infrastructure and diversity of life forms. The key to this framework is to redirect most global thoughts to local action on the micro-level so that you do not become overextended. However, a global immersion, such as a service learning experience or other fieldwork in a developing country, typically has an exponential impact when participants have a forum in which to advertise the value of the experience.

CLINICAL VOICE: AN EXEMPLAR AT THE MICRO-LEVEL

As a PhD-prepared community health nurse, I have a remarkable *pro bono* client in my private practice whom I met through a nursing student. My client, David, now age 33, has lived with locked-in syndrome for 12 years, following two traumatic brain injuries. He has given permission to tell his story as he enjoys helping others directly and indirectly.

At age 19, while changing a tire on the side of the road, David was a hit-and-run victim of a drunk driver. He survived torn spinal nerves, a skull fracture, and a 1-week coma. His treatment featured a protocol at the Mayo Clinic including nerve grafts to the cervical spine and left biceps. He recovered sufficiently to return to college.

At age 21, David sustained a grand-mal seizure and fall, undoubtedly connected to his previous injury. He endured another skull fracture, and this time his coma lasted 5 months. He awoke to paralysis of voluntary muscles from the neck down, loss of speech, and loss of vision in his right eye. He was treated for 6 months at a community hospital and nursing home, 4 months at a rehabilitation hospital, 2 years at a subacute facility where his tracheostomy was successfully closed, 5 months at an assisted living center that found his needs

CLINICAL VOICE: AN EXEMPLAR AT THE MICRO-LEVEL—cont'd

too intense for staff, and 6 years at a skilled nursing facility with minimal in-house services.

In mid-2008, at his request and with the devoted attention and help of his father, I sought community resources to improve his quality of life. A year later, David transitioned to a rented room in a wheelchair-accessible home in a quiet neighborhood, where he has lived successfully and safely for more than 4 years.

David can move his head side to side and up and down and has some control of his mouth, including the ability to smile. With his vivid blue eyes, he looks up for yes and down for no and uses an alphabet system (letter-by-letter dictation until word recognition occurs) or an electronic device, with which he scans letters and phrases to post via a switch he taps with his head. With either form of communication he is precise, organized, and articulate. He can vocalize to some extent, including laughing, which is music to my ears. He gets out of bed into a wheelchair every day via a Hoyer lift and has resumed his college studies through online instruction.

My former student went to high school with David and has been a faithful visitor ever since David's diagnosis of locked-in syndrome. In fact, my student's compassion for his friend played a major role in his pursuit of a nursing degree. After tagging along on a couple of visits with my student, I asked David, "Would you like to teach your communication methods to nursing students?" He replied via the letter-by-letter method, "Let us bargain about compensation." That was when I knew he was a person full of hopes, wishes, dreams, and good humor.

From his abiding faith, David has become unwaveringly positive, grateful, and confident. He believes "incurable" means "curable from within" and is working hard to achieve renewed goals for career, marriage, and children. Through repeated "proxy" use of his right arm to simulate feeding himself, he has regained the ability to raise and lower his forearm and remains hopeful for any additional restoration of function. Through my private practice, I consult with David and his father to facilitate evidence-based care, consultations with brain scientists and rehabilitation specialists, and updated evaluations for foundation funding. He has already received an upgraded wheelchair and computer. New interfaces have increased his communication outreach via e-mail and will eventually permit remote control of his environment, such as lighting and room temperature. With his renewed zest for living, David pursues social interaction and has met more than 1,000 students, nurses, and even U.S. President Barack Obama! This brilliant young man is inspiring on so many levels and epitomizes the reward of a micro-level investment through professional nursing.

As you consider your career path, plan a trajectory that makes sense from the following perspectives, as promoted through Campbell's Moving Mountains Self-Care Framework:

- What you love to do: If you do not know, what do you think about when you are daydreaming? Think back to your childhood. How did you spend unscheduled time?
- What you have passion for: If you do not know, what draws out indignant anger? Do you rise up against poverty, ignorance, disease, or injustice?
- What you have compassion for: If you do not know, what moves you to tears, or whose tears move you? Your compassion is a clue to the population you should serve.
- What your infrastructure or path suggests for your next step: If you do not know, chart a timeline of significant events. What have the pivotal events of your life been?
- When you live from an enduring center and express yourself through core values and deliberate action, you enhance the opportunity for clarity and deep satisfaction in your career choices. In addition, you go beyond merely balancing roles to engaging in consciously competent reflection of your most authentic self.

In the next section, we explore future roles to consider for your career path in professional nursing. We include discussion of career development strategies via mentorship. We also explain the Doctor of Nursing Practice degree, which the American Association of Colleges of Nursing has identified and endorsed as the appropriate degree for entry to advanced clinical practice.

Exploring Future Roles

We hope you remain in nursing for the balance of your career. Nursing offers a range of practice opportunities limited only by your imagination and ability to tap into resources:

- Direct patient care: Acute and chronic care in a variety of settings, including hospital, home, community agency, public health agency, long-term care, and parishes.
- Entrepreneurship: Inventive or creative approaches to deliver care, develop products, provide services, and offer consultation.
- Nursing education: Promotion of safe, competent care by preceptors, clinical scholars, clinical nurse leaders, and nurse educators in academic settings.

- Advanced practice roles: Certified clinical nurse specialists, certified registered nurse anesthetists, certified nurse midwives, and certified nurse practitioners.
- Dual roles: A simultaneous path in advanced practice and nursing education; in many settings the combination offers a "work smarter, not harder" approach to maintaining currency in advanced practice roles.

Market Your Vision for Advanced Practice During Your Graduate Program

In the late 1990s, a family nurse practitioner program graduated more than 20 students living beyond the metropolitan areas of a western state, including sparsely populated counties. Critics challenged the program director for graduating so many students at one time: "How will they ever find employment?"

In fact, all the students secured employment in advanced practice roles on graduation. Several of them established autonomous practices, and others joined existing family practices. These graduate students made a point of demonstrating their value in bringing health care to people where they live and sharing their vision for ways to increase a patient's "armamentarium," or full array of health-promoting options to every care situation, via targeted education in health promotion and disease prevention. Precepting nurse practitioners and physicians became their champions and provided recommendations, collaborative agreements, and partnerships.

Career Development

Embrace the multigenerational workforce by finding a mentor or two among long-established nurses. The best mentors are too busy to seek you out, but they enjoy working with younger or less experienced RNs. Like anyone, they are flattered by recognition and pleased when their gifts can influence others for the better. Approach potential mentors with the nursing process in mind; assess them for a good fit with your interests (Box 10–2, "A New Take on Mentorship").

Role models are powerful mentors. To that end, we provide a doctorally prepared certified nurse practitioner's view of his career trajectory. The following Clinical Voice links core values with career development and gives you a window from which to view and compare your own trajectory.

CLINICAL VOICE: CORE VALUES AND CAREER DEVELOPMENT

My nursing philosophy focuses on three aspects: competence, compassion, and caring. Competence is an important factor with which to address the current issue of evidence-based practice in nursing. If we are to care competently, we must be sure our interventions are efficacious and based on scientific rationale. Society expects nurses not only to care but also to be capable and competent in their actions.

Caring is synonymous with nursing. Although a domain definition of nursing remains elusive, I choose to define caring as simply the practice of the Golden Rule: Do to others as you would have them do to you. Caring is an essential facet, and our nursing mission should be to recognize the humanness in our patients and to care for the whole person.

Compassion is another necessary characteristic. Its etymology indicates its importance: "com" = with, and "passion" = boundless enthusiasm. As nurses we should be competent and caring and deliver our efforts with boundless enthusiasm. Competence without caring is dehumanizing, caring without competence is dangerous. Competent caring, without compassion, is to relegate our activities to a rote repetition of tasks.

My career goals remain consistent: to teach; to expand nursing knowledge; and to provide compassionate, competent care. As a nurse practitioner, I defend and promote my nursing perspective with the physician and nurse colleagues with whom I work. As a preceptor and educator, I plan to continue enlightening and empowering new graduate nurses.

Box 10–2 A New Take on Mentorship

Identify your needs or strengths (or both) for mentorship through a unique approach: review the characteristics in Gladwell's 2002 book, *The Tipping Point*:

- A maven is an "information broker" who epitomizes the "genius of the *and*" in being both a teacher and a student. A maven does not persuade but rather shares his or her own motivation to educate and help. People typically follow a maven's advice because the maven makes an emphatically convincing case. Mavens are data banks; they provide the message of the day.
- A connector knows many people and gives advice that about half the people receiving it choose to follow. A connector's importance also stems from the kind of people he or she knows. Connectors occupy multiple roles, settings, and niches, most likely because of something intrinsic

Box 10–2 A New Take on Mentorship—cont'd

to their personality, such as confidence, social skills, or personal drive. Connectors are "social glue"; they spread the message of the day.

- A salesperson is persuasive, especially in situations where some confusion persists despite available evidence. The powers of persuasion of salespeople can be subtle, such as nodding or smiling, or more overtly charismatic. They generally exude enthusiasm, love to help, and value relationships deeply. Salespeople convince others to accept the message of the day.
- Occasionally, mentors possess two of the three traits. Rarer still is the trifecta—a person who is simultaneously a maven, a connector, and a salesperson.

Identify, pursue, treasure, and honor your mentors. They will open doors you might walk past. They will grant you favors that can eliminate months of individual effort. They will make your most authentic self want to rise higher.

Adapted from Gladwell, M. (2002). *The tipping point: How little things can make a big difference.* New York: Back Bay Books.

Professional Nursing Organizations

An instant mentor source for your career trajectory comes from membership in professional nursing organizations. As an active member you will find:

- Potential mentors from among leaders as well as opportunities for leadership, especially when organizations have local chapters.
- Cutting-edge education opportunities via organizations' websites, periodic meetings, and conferences as well as opportunities to apply for scholarships for your own education and research.
- Association with colleagues who might otherwise have intimidated you because of their length of experience or well-developed résumés.
- Opportunities for renewal of your nursing practice and service that

HOW DO YOU VIEW YOUR DEDICATION TO NURSING?

Convenience
Obligation
Resolution
Devotion

Become aware of those around you who practice with minimal attention to professionalism. Become explicit about the need for devotion to professional nursing through consciously competent attention to patient safety, evidence-based practice, achievement of desired outcomes, and self-actualization.

expand your horizons and promote fulfillment of your personal framework.

You might start as a member of a committee that interests you and then watch for elections for chapter board members. Because of the Internet, many organizations value the help received from "tech-savvy" nurses regardless of their length of time in nursing. Obligations often require only a few hours a month or even a quarter. The "return on investment" can be priceless. Box 10–3 provides information on induction into nursing's honor society, *Sigma Theta Tau* International.

Doctor of Nursing Practice

As you contemplate your future in nursing, we want you to be aware of and plan for a recommended evolution of advanced practice registered nurse (APRN) roles. In October 2004, the American Association of Colleges of Nursing (AACN) endorsed a document titled the *Position*

Box 10–3 Induction Into Nursing's Honor Society

Do you have your heart set on membership in the prestigious *Sigma Theta Tau* International (STTI) Honor Society of Nursing? Assuming your undergraduate program has an affiliation to STTI, the main criteria to receive an invitation to join are:

- Undergraduate GPA 3.0 and higher
- Half of all program credits completed by induction date
- Top 35% of class or cohort

Many students exceed the GPA requirement, but only the top 35% receive an invitation. For some cohorts, a GPA of 3.8 or higher may be necessary. Students who miss this cut have two more opportunities for induction:

- As a graduate student: If (more likely, when) you go to graduate school, all students with a graduate GPA 3.5 and above are invited to join after they have completed at least one quarter of their program.
- As a community nurse leader: A current STTI member can nominate RNs with a minimum of a BSN degree and demonstrated achievements in practice, administration, publishing, or education (staff, student, or patient). Some RNs self-nominate through the international headquarters, but this approach might interfere with perceiving you as a community nurse leader. If you truly do not know a chapter member to sponsor you, contact the chair of the membership committee or even the chapter president for guidance.

Data from *Sigma Theta Tau* International Honor Society of Nursing, http://www.nursingsociety.org/

Statement on the Practice Doctorate in Nursing that called for moving the level of preparation necessary for advanced nursing from the master's degree to the doctorate level by 2015. The following talking points, reproduced here with permission of the AACN, help explain this step forward for nursing education:

Doctor of Nursing Practice Degree
The Need for Change in Graduate Nursing Education

- The changing demands of the nation's complex health care environment require nurses serving in specialty positions to have the highest level of scientific knowledge and practice expertise possible. Research from Drs. Linda Aiken, Carole Estabrooks, and others have established a clear link between higher levels of nursing education and better patient outcomes.
- Key factors building momentum for change in nursing education at the graduate level include the rapid expansion of knowledge underlying practice; increased complexity of patient care; national concerns about the quality of care and patient safety; shortages of nursing personnel, which demands a higher level of preparation for leaders who can design and assess care; shortages of doctorally prepared nursing faculty; and increasing educational expectations for the preparation of other health professionals.
- The Institute of Medicine, Joint Commission, and other authorities have called for reconceptualizing health professions education to meet the needs of the health care delivery system. Nursing is answering that call by moving to prepare APRNs for evolving practice.
- In a 2005 report titled *Advancing the Nation's Health Needs: NIH Research Training Programs*, the National Academy of Sciences called for nursing to develop a non-research clinical doctorate to prepare expert practitioners who can also serve as clinical faculty. AACN's work to advance the DNP is consistent with this call to action.
- Nursing is moving in the direction of other health professions in the transition to the DNP. Medicine (MD), Dentistry (DDS), Pharmacy (PharmD), Psychology (PsyD), Physical Therapy (DPT), and Audiology (AudD) all offer practice doctorates.

Impact on Nursing Education and Practice

- Currently, APRNs—including Certified Nurse Practitioners, Certified Clinical Nurse Specialists, Certified Nurse Midwives, and Certified Registered Nurse Anesthetists—are typically prepared in master's degree programs, some of which carry a credit load equivalent to doctoral degrees in the other health professions.

- DNP curricula build on current master's programs by providing education in evidence-based practice, quality improvement, and systems thinking, among other key areas.
- Transitioning to the DNP supports APRN's achievement of full practice authority. State Nurse Practice Acts describe the scope of practice allowed, which differs from state to state. The transition to the DNP will better prepare APRNs for their current roles given the calls for new models of education and the growing complexity of health care.
- The DNP is designed for nurses seeking a terminal degree in nursing practice and offers an alternative to research-focused doctoral programs. DNP-prepared nurses will be well-equipped to fully implement the science developed by nurse researchers prepared in PhD and other research-focused nursing doctorates.
- The title of "doctor" is common to many disciplines and is not the domain of any one health profession. Many APRNs currently hold doctoral degrees and are addressed as "doctor," which is similar to how clinical psychologists, dentists, podiatrists, and other experts are addressed. Like other providers, DNPs would be expected to display their credentials to ensure that patients understand their preparation as a nursing provider.
- Nursing and medicine are distinct health disciplines that prepare clinicians to assume different roles and meet different practice expectations. DNP programs will prepare nurses for the highest level of nursing practice.

Continuing the Push for Nursing Excellence

The primary power of nursing lies in nurses' stewardship of holistic human health and healing. This comprehensive capability begs a relational journey with recipients of care to determine what constitutes "holistic" for individuals, families, groups, and communities. The pursuit of holism brings astonishing access to those recipients from birth to death. This broad spectrum of care across the life span demands that nurses bring an "armamentarium" or full array of health-promoting options to every care situation.

A Metaphor for Nursing

One way to capture the depth and breadth of nursing is to reflect on the metaphor shown in Figures 10–2 and 10–3. Figure 10–2 shows a glass with liquid at the halfway point. A familiar question is, "How would you describe this image?" Answers usually include:

- The glass is half full, which is an optimistic appraisal
- The glass is half empty, which is a pessimistic appraisal.
- The glass is too big for its contents, which is a pragmatic response.

As a metaphor for the nursing profession, the ideal answer is, "The glass is full" . . . of potential! Nurses have the power to illuminate "potential" as

HALF FULL OR HALF EMPTY?

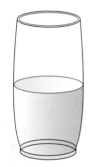

FIGURE 10–2: A metaphor for professional nursing.

Your "worldview" is important!

It's FULL

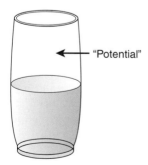

◄— "Potential"

FIGURE 10–3: Completing the metaphor for professional nursing.

they journey with patients walking every path of life, living with every health and illness state, or dying from acute or chronic conditions.

Just as powerful, nurses also take a sacred journey, the most poignant ones accompanying a patient's premature death. Typically, the nurse is the privileged lifeline for overwhelmed and grieving family members and sometimes groups or communities. Consider your patients' needs in the context of Covey's list of four needs:

- To live: The young man recovering from devastating injuries sustained in a hit-and-run accident
- To love: The young mother giving birth to healthy twins
- To learn: The middle-aged man with metabolic syndrome
- To leave a legacy: The older woman who has received a diagnosis of lung cancer with widespread metastasis

In the final section, we offer five "pearls of wisdom." These pearls constitute the advice our students have told us benefited them the most, often years later.

Pearls of Wisdom

- Work smarter, not harder: Look for a win-win outcome as often as possible. For example, if your unit requires multiple certifications from you, such as Advanced Cardiac Life Support, Trauma Nurse Core Curriculum, and Pediatric Advanced Life Support, pursue them as close together in your first year of practice as you can. Content from one course reinforces and sometimes duplicates content from another course. You also will command greater respect as an RN when you can document or validate your expanding knowledge base.
- Compile a repertoire that helps define you. Select favorite quotations, principles, and resources as you progress in your career. Develop a personal motto and brand. Track the writings of two or three inspirational nursing leaders. Attend presentations whenever possible for greater personal impact. A few words of encouragement from a nursing leader can be life-changing. Type your conference session notes, and review them from time to time. Share persistently resonating themes with your nursing network. Be friendly!
- Develop a council of advisors, and rotate members according to their ability not only to bring clarity to an issue but also to help you find *your* voice. When you have a big decision to make, consult with at least five others until your viewpoint becomes clear.

Many newer RNs make hasty decisions in the first couple of years of practice, including abandoning their nursing career, because they neglect to obtain these clarifying perspectives.

- Go where you are valued. People often have a stubborn attachment to an unconscious or unexamined notion. We have seen former students tolerate the intolerable out of misguided loyalty, insufficient information about mobility within professional nursing, or underestimation of their own abilities.
- Adopt Ruiz's articulation of "The Four Agreements": Be impeccable with your word, do not take anything personally (because both praise and criticism say more about the giver than the recipient), do not make assumptions, and always do your best. Increase your personal accountability: Cheerfully meet expectations you willingly agreed to or allowed.

As you sense you have become consciously competent, stretch more and more. Consider how you can become consciously capable. Identify the resources needed for daily excellence. Persevere until you can say with professional pride, "Mission accomplished!"

Chapter Summary

This final chapter brings you tried and true approaches for self-care and career development as you contemplate your next steps in professional nursing. We hope you will re-read this chapter whenever you need some encouragement to move forward on your path to personal and professional fulfillment. We are delighted and affirmed as we envision your pursuit of nursing excellence on behalf of recipients of care in every setting imaginable!

REFERENCES

Preface

Benner, P. (2001). *From novice to expert: Excellence and power in clinical nursing practice* (commemorative ed.). Upper Saddle River, NJ: Prentice Hall.

Covey, S. (1989). *The seven habits of highly effective people: Restoring the character ethic.* New York, NY: Simon & Schuster.

Disch, J. (2012). QSEN? What's QSEN? *Nursing Outlook, 60*(2), 58–59.

Goode, C. (2000). What constitutes the "evidence" in evidence-based practice? *Applied Nursing Research, 13*(4), 222–225.

Grbach, W. (2007). Teaching strategies: Reformulating SBAR to "I-SBAR-R." Retrieved from http://qsen.org/?s = I-SBAR-R

Greenleaf, R. K. (2002). *Servant Leadership: A journey into the nature of legitimate power and greatness* (25th anniversary ed.). Mahwah, NJ: Paulist Press.

Peters, T. (1999). *The circle of innovation: You can't shrink your way to greatness.* New York, NY: Vintage Books.

Russo, G. (2007, 14 June). In search of the super-mentor. *Nature, 447*, 881.

Yancer, D. A. (2012). Betrayed trust: Healing a broken hospital through Servant Leadership. *Nursing Administration Quarterly, 36*(1), 63–80.

Chapter 1: Providing a Framework to Accelerate Your Transition to Practicing RN

American Nurses Association. (2010). *Nursing: Scope and standards of practice* (2nd ed.). Silver Spring, MD: nursesbooks.org

Benner, P. (2001). *From novice to expert: Excellence and power in clinical nursing practice* (Commemorative ed.). Upper Saddle River, NJ: Prentice Hall.

Berkow, S., Virkstis, K., Stewart, J., & Conway, L. (2008). Assessing new graduate nurse performance. *The Journal of Nursing Administration, 38*(11), 468–474.

Casey, K., Fink, R., Jaynes, C., Campbell, L., Cook, P., & Wilson, V. (2011). Readiness for practice: The senior practicum experience. *Journal of Nursing Education, 50*, 646–652. doi: 10.3928/01484834-20110817-03

Casey, K., Fink, R., Krugman, M., & Propst, J. (2004). The graduate nurse experience. *Journal of Nursing Administration, 34*(6), 303–311.

Collins, J. C., & Porras, J. I. (1997). *Built to last: Successful habits of visionary companies.* New York, NY: HarperCollins.

Covey, S. (1989). *The seven habits of highly effective people: Restoring the character ethic.* New York, NY: Simon & Schuster.

Cronenwett, L., Sherwood, G., Barnsteiner, J., Disch, J., et al. (2007). Quality and safety education for nurses. *Nursing Outlook, 55*, 122–131.

Disch, J. (2012). QSEN? What's QSEN? *Nursing Outlook, 60*(2), 58–59.

Goode, C. (2000). What constitutes the "evidence" in evidence-based practice? *Applied Nursing Research, 13*(4), 222–225.

Greenleaf, R. K. (2002). *Servant Leadership: A journey into the nature of legitimate power and greatness* (25th anniversary ed.). Mahwah, NJ: Paulist Press.

Hopp, L., & Rittenmeyer, L. (2012). *Introduction to evidence-based practice: A practical guide for nursing.* Philadelphia, PA: F. A. Davis.

Peters, T. (1999). *The circle of innovation: You can't shrink your way to greatness.* New York, NY: Vintage Books.

Steen, J. E., Gould, E. W., Raingruber, B., & Hill, J. (2011). Effect of student nurse intern position on ease of transition from student nurse to Registered Nurse. *Journal for Nurses in Staff Development, 27*(4), 181–186.

Swanson, K. M. (1990). Providing care in the NICU: Sometimes an act of love. *Advances in Nursing Science, 13*(1), 60–73.

Tahan, H. A. (2004). Leader to watch: Daniel J. Pesut, APRN, BC, PhD, FAAN: A creative thinker and futuristic leader. *Nurse Leader, 2*(3), 10–14.

Tilden, V. P., & Tilden, S. (2011, Wiley Online Publication). *From novice to expert, excellence and power in clinical nursing practice.* (Book Review). *Research in Nursing & Health, 8*, 95–97. doi: 10.1002/nur.4770080119

Washington, G. T. (2012). Performance anxiety in new graduate nurses: Is it for real? *Dimensions of Critical Care Nursing, 31*, 295–300. doi: 10.1097/DCC.0b013e3182619b4c

Yancer, D. A. (2012). Betrayed trust: Healing a broken hospital through Servant Leadership. *Nursing Administration Quarterly, 36*(1), 63–80.

Chapter 2: Pathophysiology and Pharmacology: Making Connections and Mastering Dosage Calculations

American Diabetes Association. (2013). Summary of revisions for the 2013 Clinical Practice Recommendations. *Diabetes Care, 36*, S3. doi: 10.2337/dc13-S003

American Diabetes Association. (2011). *National diabetes fact sheet.* Alexandria, VA: American Diabetes Association.

Amorim, M. M. R., Souza, A. S. R., Katz, L., & Noronha Neto, C. (2011). Planned caesarean section versus planned vaginal delivery for severe preeclampsia (Protocol). *Cochrane Database of Systematic Reviews 2011*, Issue 11. Art. No.: CD009430. doi: 10.1002/14651858.CD009430

Burr, J., Azuara-Blanco, A., Avenell, A., & Tuulonen, A. (2012). Medical versus surgical interventions for open angle glaucoma. *Cochrane Database of Systematic Reviews 2012*, Issue 9. Art. No.: CD004399. doi: 10.1002/14651858.CD004399.pub3

Callaghan, B. C., Little, A. A., Feldman, E. L., & Hughes, R. A. C. (2012). Enhanced glucose control for preventing and treating diabetic neuropathy. *Cochrane Database of Systematic Reviews 2012*, Issue 6. Art. No.: CD007543. doi: 10.1002/14651858.CD007543.pub2

Chey, W. D., & Wong, B. C. Y. (2007). American College of Gastroenterology guideline on the management of *Helicobacter pylori* infection. *American Journal of Gastroenterology, 102*, 1808–1825. doi: 10.1111/j.1572-0241.2007.01393.x

Davies, E. J., Moxham, T., Rees, K., Singh, S., Coats, A. J. S., Ebrahim, S., . . . Taylor, R. S. (2010). Exercise based rehabilitation for heart failure. *Cochrane*

Database of Systematic Reviews 2010, Issue 4. Art. No.: CD003331. doi: 10.1002/14651858.CD003331.pub3

DeVault, K. R., & Castell, D. O. (2005). Updated guidelines for the diagnosis and treatment of gastroesophageal reflux disease. *American Journal of Gastroenterology, 100,* 190–200.

Elward, K. S., & Pollart, S. M. (2010, Nov. 15). Medical therapy for asthma: Updates from the NAEPP Guidelines. *American Family Physician, 82*(10), 1242–1251.

Faris, R. F., Flather, M., Purcell, H., Poole-Wilson, P. A., & Coats, A. J. S. (2012). Diuretics for heart failure. *Cochrane Database of Systematic Reviews 2012,* Issue 2. Art. No.: CD003838. doi: 10.1002/14651858.CD003838.pub3

Fendrick, A. M., Forsch, R. T., Van Harrison, R., & Scheiman, J. M. (2005). *Guidelines for Clinical Care—Peptic ulcer disease.* Retrieved from University of Michigan Health System Ann Arbor Web site: http://www.med.umich.edu

Fingeret, M. (2011). *Optometric Clinical Practice Guideline care of the patient with open angle glaucoma.* St. Louis, MO: American Optometric Association.

Ford, A. C., Delaney, B., Forman, D., & Moayyedi, P. (2011 [updated]). Eradication therapy for peptic ulcer disease in *Helicobacter pylori* positive patients. Original publication: *Cochrane Database of Systematic Reviews 2006,* Issue 2. Art. No.: CD003840. doi: 10.1002/14651858.CD003840.pub4

Greener, M. (2011). Easing the burden of COPD: NICE guidelines and new agents. *Nurse Prescribing, 9*(2), 64–67.

Greenfield, S., Whelan, B., & Cohn, E. (2006). Use of dimensional analysis to reduce medication errors. *Journal of Nursing Education, 45,* 91–94.

Heran, B. S., Musini, V. M., Bassett, K., Taylor, R. S., & Wright, J. M. (2012). Angiotensin receptor blockers for heart failure. *Cochrane Database of Systematic Reviews 2012,* Issue 4. Art. No.: CD003040. doi: 10.1002/14651858.CD003040.pub2

Hunt, S. A., Abraham, W. T., Chin, M. H., Feldman, A. M., Francis, G. S., Ganiats, T. G., . . . Yancy, C. W. (2009). 2009 focused update incorporated into the ACC/AHA 2005 Guidelines for the Diagnosis and Management of Heart Failure in Adults. *Circulation, 119,* e391–e479.

Iley, K. (2012). Improving palliative care for patients with COPD. *Nursing Standard, 26,* 37, 40–46.

Karner, C., & Cates, C. J. (2012). Long-acting beta$_2$-agonist in addition to tiotropium versus either tiotropium or long-acting beta$_2$-agonist alone for chronic obstructive pulmonary disease. *Cochrane Database of Systematic Reviews 2012,* Issue 4. Art. No.: CD008989. doi: 10.1002/14651858.CD008989.pub2

Lagerquist, S. L. (ed.). (2012). *Davis's NCLEX-RN success* (3rd ed.). Philadelphia, PA: F. A. Davis.

Lambert, M. (2012, Apr 15). NICE updates guidelines on management of chronic heart failure. *American Family Physician, 85*(8), 832–834.

Lehne, R. A. (2010). *Pharmacology for nursing care* (7th ed.). St. Louis, MO: Saunders.

Leyshon, J. (2012). Managing severe breathlessness in patients with end-stage COPD. *Nursing Standard, 27*(6), 48–56.

Lip, G. Y. H., Wrigley, B. J., & Pisters, R. (2012). Anticoagulation versus placebo for heart failure in sinus rhythm. *Cochrane Database of Systematic Reviews 2012,* Issue 6. Art. No.: CD003336. doi: 10.1002/14651858.CD003336.pub2

Malanda, U. L., Welschen, L. M. C., Riphagen, I. I., Dekker, J. M., Nijpels, G., & Bot, S. D. M. (2012). Self-monitoring of blood glucose in patients with type 2 diabetes mellitus who are not using insulin. *Cochrane Database of Systematic Reviews 2012,* Issue 1. Art. No.: CD005060. doi: 10.1002/14651858. CD005060.pub3

Marsh, K., Barclay, A., Colagiuri, S., & Brand-Miller, J. (2011). Glycemic index and glycemic load of carbohydrates in the diabetes diet. *Current Diabetes Reports, 11,* 120–127. doi: 10.1007/s11892-010-0173-8

McCance, K. L., & Huether, S. E. (2010). *Pathophysiology: The biologic basis for disease in adults and children* (6th ed.). St. Louis, MO: Mosby.

Moayyedi, P., Santana, J., Khan, M., Preston, C., & Donnellan, C. (2011). Medical treatments in the short term management of reflux oesophagitis. *Cochrane Database of Systematic Reviews 2011,* Issue 2. Art. No.: CD003244. doi: 10.1002/14651858.CD003244.pub3

National Council of State Boards of Nursing. (2013). NCLEX-RN test plan. Retrieved from https://www.ncsbn.org/2013_NCLEX_RN_Detailed_Test_Plan_Candidate.pdf

National Guideline Clearinghouse. (2005, Mar). Registered Nurses Association of Ontario (RNAO). *Nursing care of dyspnea: The 6th vital sign in individuals with chronic obstructive pulmonary disease (COPD).* Retrieved from http://www. guideline.gov/content.aspx?id = 32419&search = dyspnea

National Guideline Clearinghouse. (2000, Sept; revised 2010). American Academy of Ophthalmology Glaucoma Panel, Preferred Practice Patterns Committee (2010). *Primary angle closure.* Retrieved from http://www.guideline.gov/ content.aspx?id = 24812&search = glaucoma + and + primary + angle + closure

National Guideline Clearinghouse. (1995, revised 2002, Aug; reviewed 2007; revised 2010). *American Optometric Association: Care of the patient with open angle glaucoma* (2nd ed.). Retrieved from http://www.guideline.gov/content. aspx?id = 33582&search = open + angle + glaucoma

National Heart, Lung and Blood Institute. (Revised 2007, Aug). *National Heart, Lung and Blood Institute/National Asthma Education and Prevention Program (NAEPP) Expert Panel Report 3: Guidelines for the Diagnosis and Management of Asthma (EPR-3).* Retrieved from http://www.nhlbi.nih.gov/guidelines/asthma/ asthgdln.pdf

Pogson, Z., & McKeever, T. (2011). Dietary sodium manipulation and asthma. *Cochrane Database of Systematic Reviews 2011,* Issue 3. Art. No.: CD000436. doi: 10.1002/14651858.CD000436.pub3

Poole, P., Black, P. N., & Cates, C. J. (2012). Mucolytic agents for chronic bronchitis or chronic obstructive pulmonary disease. *Cochrane Database of*

Systematic Reviews 2012, Issue 8. Art. No.: CD001287. doi: 10.1002/14651858. CD001287.pub4

Stoloff, S. W., & Kelly, H. W. (2011). Updates on the use of inhaled corticosteroids in asthma. *Current Opinion in Allergy & Clinical Immunology, 11*(4), 337–344.

Tang, R. S., & Chan, F. K. L. (2012). Therapeutic management of recurrent peptic ulcer disease. *Drugs, 72*(12), 1605–1616.

Twedell, D. (2009). Symptom check: Is it GERD? *The Journal of Continuing Education in Nursing, 40*(3), 103–104.

Vallerand, A. H., & Sanoski, C. A. (2013). *Davis's drug guide for nurses* (13th ed.). Philadelphia, PA: F. A. Davis.

Van Leeuwen, A. M., Poelhuis-Leth, D., & Bladh, M. L. (2011). *Davis's comprehensive handbook of laboratory and diagnostic tests with nursing implications* (4th ed.). Philadelphia, PA: F. A. Davis.

Wilkinson, J. M., & Treas, L. S. (2011). *Procedure checklists for fundamentals of nursing* (2nd ed.). Philadelphia, PA: F. A. Davis.

World Health Organization. (2011). *WHO recommendations for prevention and treatment of pre-eclampsia and eclampsia*. Geneva, Switzerland: WHO. Retrieved from http://whqlibdoc.who.int/publications/2011/9789241548335_eng.pdf

Chapter 3: Physical Assessment Skills and Findings: Firming the Foundation of Nursing Process

Dillon, P. (2007). *Nursing health assessment: A critical thinking case studies approach.* Philadelphia, PA: F. A. Davis.

Jarvis, C. (2012). *Physical examination and health assessment* (6th ed.). St. Louis, MO: Saunders.

McEwen, D., & Dumpel, H. (2011). HIPAA—the Health Insurance Portability and Accountability Act: What RNs need to know about privacy rules and protected health information. *National Nurse, 107*(7), 18–26.

News and innovation. (2012). *Journal of Pain & Palliative Care Pharmacotherapy, 26*, 204–212.

Spade, C. M. (2008). Psychosocial vital signs: Using simulation to introduce a new concept. *Nurse Educator, 33*(4), 181–186.

Spade, C. M., & Mulhall, M. (2010). Teaching psychosocial vital signs across the undergraduate nursing curriculum. *Clinical Simulation in Nursing, 6*, e143–e151. doi: 10.1016/j.ecns.2009.10.002

U.S. Department of Health and Human Services. (2013). *Understanding health information privacy.* Washington, DC: Author. Retrieved from http://www.hhs.gov/ocr/privacy/hipaa/understanding/index.html

U.S. Department of Health and Human Services. (2013). *Breach notification rule.* Washington, DC: Author. Retrieved from http://www.hhs.gov/ocr/privacy/hipaa/administrative/breachnotificationrule/

Chapter 4: Diagnostics: Understanding and Monitoring Common Laboratory Tests

Aziz, A. (2011). Audit of blood culture technique and documentation to improve practice. *British Journal of Nursing, (Intravenous Supplement), 20*(8), S26–S34.

Barnette, L., & Kautz, D. (2013). Creative ways to teach arterial blood gas interpretation. *Dimensions of Critical Care Nursing, 32*(2), 84–87.

Casey, K., Fink, R., Krugman, M., & Propst, J. (2004). The graduate nurse experience. *Journal of Nursing Administration, 34*(6), 303–311.

Dexter, F., Ledolter, J., Davis, E., Witkowski, T. A., Herman, J. H., Epstein, R. H. (2012). Systematic criteria for type and screen based on procedure's probability of erythrocyte transfusion. *Anesthesiology, 116*(4), 768–778.

Dubin, D. (2000). *Rapid interpretation of EKGs* (6th ed.). Fort Myers, FL: COVER Publishing.

Fischbach, F. T., & Dunning, M. B. (2009). *A manual of laboratory and diagnostic tests* (8th ed.). Philadelphia, PA: Lippincott Williams & Wilkins.

Huff, J. (2012). *ECG workout: Exercises in arrhythmia interpretation* (6th ed.). Ambler, PA: Lippincott Williams, & Wilkins.

Jones, S. A. (2009). *ECG notes: Interpretation and management guide* (2nd ed.). Philadelphia, PA: F. A. Davis.

Karch, A. M, (2012). Pharmacology review: Drugs that alter blood coagulation. *American Nurse Today, 7*(11), 26–30.

Pagana, K. D., & Pagana, T. (2010) *Mosby's manual of diagnostic and laboratory tests* (4th ed.). St. Louis, MO: Mosby.

Potter, P. A., & Perry, A. G. (2013). *Fundamentals of nursing* (8th ed.). St. Louis, MO: Mosby.

Rowley, S., & Clare, S. (2011). ANTT: an essential tool for effective blood culture collection. *British Journal of Nursing, (Intravenous Supplement), 20*(14), S9–S14.

Van Leeuwen, A. M., Poelhuis-Leth, D., & Bladh, M. L. (2011). *Davis's comprehensive handbook of laboratory and diagnostic tests with nursing implications* (4th ed.). Philadelphia, PA: F. A. Davis.

Venes, D. (ed.). (2013). *Taber's cyclopedic medical dictionary* (22nd ed.). Philadelphia, PA: F. A. Davis.

Vonfrolio, L. G. (2008). *The ABCs of ABGs*. Staten Island, NY: Education Enterprises. Available from www.greatnurses.com

Chapter 5: Patient Care: Reviewing Critical Skills, Keeping Patients Safe, and Managing Machines

Alekseyev, S., Byrne, M., Carpenter, A., Franker, C., Kidd, C., & Hulton, L. (2012). Prolonging the life of a patient's IV: An integrative review of intravenous securement devices. *MEDSURG Nursing, 21*(5), 285–292.

Apelseth, T. O., Molnar, L., Arnold, E., & Heddle, N. M. (2012). Benchmarking: Applications to transfusion medicine. *Transfusion Medicine Reviews, 26*(4), 321–332.

Bard Medical. (2013). Advance: Foley tray system directions for use. Covington, GA: Author. Retrieved from http://m.bardmedical.com/media/2952/Advance%20DFU%20Poster.pdf

Bard Medical. (2013). Bard Foley Catheter inflation/deflation guidelines. Covington, GA: Author. Retrieved from http://bardmedical.com/Resources/Products/Documents/Brochures/Urology/FoleyInflationDeflationGuidelines.pdf

Best, C. (2007). Nasogastric tube insertion in adults who require enteral feeding. *Nursing Standard 2007, 21*(40), 39–43.

Casey, K., Fink, R., Jaynes, C., Campbell, L., Cook, P., & Wilson, V. (2011). Readiness for practice: The senior practicum experience. *Journal of Nursing Education, 50*, 646–652. doi: 10.3928/01484834-20110817-03

Cengiz, E., Swan, K. L., Tamborlane, W. V., Sherr, J. L., Martin, M., & Weinzimer, S. A. (2012). The alteration of aspart insulin pharmacodynamics when mixed with detemir insulin. *Diabetes Care, 35*(4), 690–692.

Cengiz, E., Tamborlane, W. V., Martin-Fredericksen, M., Dziura, J., & Weinzimer, S. A. (2010). Early pharmacokinetic and pharmacodynamic effects of mixing lispro with glargine insulin: Results of glucose clamp studies in youth with type 1 diabetes. *Diabetes Care, 33*(5), 1009–1012.

Centers for Disease Control and Prevention. (2011). Guidelines for the prevention of intravascular catheter-related infections, 2011. Retrieved from http://www.cdc.gov/hicpac/pdf/guidelines/bsi-guidelines-2011.pdf

Centers for Disease Control and Prevention. (n.d.). National Health and Nutrition Examination Survey III: Electrocardiogram. Retrieved from http://www.cdc.gov/nchs/data/nhanes/nhanes3/cdrom/nchs/manuals/ecg.pdf

Chenoweth, C., & Saint, S. (2013). Preventing catheter-associated urinary tract infections in the intensive care unit. *Critical Care Clinics, 29*(1), 19–32.

Dinter, T. G. V., John, L., Guileyardo, J. M., & Fordtran, J. S. (2013). Intestinal perforation caused by insertion of a nasogastric tube late after gastric bypass. *Baylor University Medical Center Proceedings, 26*(1), 11–15.

Dokken, B. B. (2013). How insulin analogues can benefit patients. *The Nurse Practitioner, 38*(2), 44–48.

Freeman, D., Saxton, V., & Holberton, J. (2012). A weight-based formula for the estimation of gastric tube insertion length in newborns. *Advances in Neonatal Care, 12*(3), 179–182.

Henneman, E. A., Gawlinski, A., & Giuliano, K. K. (2012). Surveillance: A strategy for improving patient safety in acute and critical care units. *Critical Care Nurse, 32*(2), e9–e18.

Infusion Nurses Society. (2011). Infusion nursing standards of practice. *Journal of Infusion Nursing, 54*(1S), S46–S47.

Laustsen, G. (2005). Finely honed nursing skills. In S. Hudacek (Ed.), *Making a difference: Stories from the point of care* (Vol. 1, pp. 173–174). Indianapolis, IN: *Sigma Theta Tau* International.

Lynn, P. (2011). *Taylor's clinical nursing skills: A nursing process approach* (3rd ed.). Philadelphia, PA: Lippincott Williams & Wilkins.

Madias, J. E. (2011). Why recording of an electrocardiogram should be required in every inpatient and outpatient encounter of patients with heart failure. *Pacing & Clinical Electrophysiology, 34*(8), 963–967.

Melendez, L., & Pino, R. M. (2012). Electrocardiogram interference: a thing of the past? *Biomedical Instrumentation & Technology, 46*(6), 470–477.

MPR. (2012–13). Insulin administration. In *Nurse practitioners' prescribing reference*. New York, NY: Author.

Naccarato, M., Leviner, S., Proehl, J., Barnason, S., Brim, C., Crowley, M., . . . Papa, A. M. (2012). Emergency nursing resource: Orthostatic vital signs. *Journal of Emergency Nursing, 38*, 447–453. doi: 10.1016/j.jen.2012.05.011

Phillips, L. D. (2010). *Manual of I.V. therapeutics* (5th ed.). Philadelphia, PA: F. A. Davis.

St. Clair, J. (2005). A new model of tracheostomy care: Closing the research-practice gap. Retrieved from http://www.ahrq.gov/downloads/pub/advances/vol3/Clair.pdf

St. John, R. E., & Malen, J. F. (2004). Contemporary issues in adult tracheostomy management. *Critical Care Nursing Clinics of North America, 16*(3), 413–430.

Turkel, M. C., Ray, M. A., & Kornblatt, L. (2012). Instead of reconceptualizing the Nursing Process, let's re-name it. *Nursing Science Quarterly, 25*(2), 194–198.

van Tulder, R., Roth, D., Weiser, C., Heidinger, B., Herkner, H., Schreiber W., & Havel, C. (2012). An electrocardiogram technician improves in-hospital first medical contact-to-electrocardiogram times: a cluster randomized controlled interventional trial. *American Journal of Emergency Medicine, 30*(9), 1729–1736.

Venes, D. (ed.). (2013). *Taber's cyclopedic medical dictionary* (22nd ed.). Philadelphia, PA: F. A. Davis.

Westgard, E. (2011). *Clinical coach for fluid & electrolyte balance*. Philadelphia, PA: F. A. Davis.

Wilkinson, J. M., & Treas, L. S. (2011). *Procedure checklists for fundamentals of nursing* (2nd ed.). Philadelphia, PA: F. A. Davis.

Chapter 6: Shift Planning: Conquering Shift Organization and Prioritization

Agency for Healthcare Research and Quality (AHRQ). (2011). Patient safety primers: Never events. Retrieved from http://www.psnet.ahrq.gov/primer.aspx?primerID=3

Byrne, R. (2006). *The secret*. New York, NY: Simon & Schuster.

Castillo, S. L. (2009). *Strategies, techniques, and approaches to thinking: Critical thinking cases in nursing* (4th ed.). St. Louis, MO: Saunders.

Dillon, P. (2007). *Nursing health assessment: A critical thinking case studies approach*. Philadelphia, PA: F. A. Davis.

Doenges, M. E., Moorhouse, M. F., & Murr, A. C. (2010). *Nurse's pocket guide: Diagnoses, prioritized interventions, and rationales* (12th ed.). Philadelphia, PA: F. A. Davis.

Joint Commission. (2012). Sentinel event policy and procedures. Retrieved from http://www.jointcommission.org/Sentinel_Event_Policy_and_Procedures/

McCance, K. L., & Huether, S. E. (2010). *Pathophysiology: The biologic basis for disease in adults and children* (6th ed.). St. Louis, MO: Mosby.

Novak, K., & Fairchild, R. (2012). Bedside reporting and SBAR: Improving patient communication and satisfaction. *Journal of Pediatric Nursing, 27*(6), 760–762.

Solari-Twadell, P. A., Bunkers, S. S., Wang, C., & Snyder, D. (1995). The pinwheel model of bereavement. *Journal of Nursing Scholarship, 27*(4), 323–326.

Spade, C. M., & Mulhall, M. (2010). Teaching psychosocial vital signs across the undergraduate nursing curriculum. *Clinical Simulation in Nursing, 6*, e143–e151. doi: 10.1016/j.ecns.2009.10.002

Van Leeuwen, A. M., Poelhuis-Leth, D., & Bladh, M. L. (2011). *Davis's comprehensive handbook of laboratory and diagnostic tests with nursing implications* (4th ed.). Philadelphia, PA: F. A. Davis.

Wilkinson, J. M., & Treas, L. S. (2011). *Procedure checklists for fundamentals of nursing* (2nd ed.). Philadelphia, PA: F. A. Davis.

Chapter 7: Communication: Mastering Collaboration, Delegation, and Documentation

Compton, J., Copeland, K., Flanders, S., Cassity, C., Spetman, M., Xiao, Y., & Kennerly, D. (2012). Implementing SBAR across a large multihospital health system. *Joint Commission Journal on Quality & Patient Safety, 38*(6), 261–268.

Dillon, P. (2007). *Nursing health assessment: A critical thinking case studies approach.* Philadelphia, PA: F. A. Davis.

Doenges, M. E., Moorhouse, M. F., & Murr, A. C. (2010). *Nurse's pocket guide: Diagnoses, prioritized interventions, and rationales* (12th ed.). Philadelphia: F. A. Davis.

Grbach, W. (2007). Teaching strategies: *Reformulating SBAR to "I-SBAR-R."* Retrieved from http://qsen.org/?s=I-SBAR-R

Halldorsdottir, S. (1991). Five basic modes of being with another. In D. Gaut & M. M. Leininger (Eds.), *Caring: The compassionate healer* (pp. 37–49). New York, NY: National League for Nursing.

Joint Commission. (2013). *National patient safety goals.* Oakbrook Terrace, IL: Author. Retrieved from http://www.jointcommission.org/standards_information/npsgs.aspx

Joint Commission. (2013). *Facts about the official list of "do not use" abbreviations.* Oakbrook Terrace, IL: Author. Retrieved from http://www.jointcommission.org/standards_information/npsgs.aspx

LaCharity, L. A., Kumagai, C. K., & Bartz, B. (2011). *Prioritization, delegation, & assignment: Practice exercises for medical-surgical nursing* (2nd ed.). St. Louis, MO: Mosby.

Marill, M. (2013). Joint Commission: You can't have patient safety without HCW safety. *Hospital Employee Health, 32*(1), 1–3.

Mehl, M. R., Vazire, S., Ramirez-Esparza, N., Statcher, R. B., et al. (2007, July). Are women really more talkative than men? *Science, 317,* 82.

National Council of State Boards of Nursing and American Nurses Association. (2006, September 12). *Joint statement on delegation.* Retrieved from https://www.ncsbn.org/Delegation_joint_statement_NCSBN-ANA.pdf

Newland, J. A. (2013). The advantages of being multilingual. *The Nurse Practitioner, 38*(2), 5.

SBAR Technique for Communication: A situational briefing model. (2011). Retrieved from Institute for Healthcare Improvement Web site: http://www.ihi.org/knowledge/Pages/Tools/SBARTechniqueforCommunicationASituational BriefingModel.aspx

Sherman, R. O. (2006). Leading a multigenerational nursing workforce: Issues, challenges and strategies. *Online Journal of Issues in Nursing, 11*(2), 5 pages.

Sparks, A. M. (2012). Psychological empowerment and job satisfaction between Baby Boomer and Generation X nurses. *Journal of Nursing Management, 20,* 451–460. doi: 10.1111/j.1365-2834.2011.01282.x

Van Leeuwen, A. M., Poelhuis-Leth, D., & Bladh, M. L. (2011). *Davis's comprehensive handbook of laboratory and diagnostic tests with nursing implications* (4th ed.). Philadelphia, PA: F. A. Davis.

Venes, D. (Ed.). (2013). The interpreter in three languages. In *Taber's Cyclopedic Medical Dictionary* (22nd ed., Appendix 8). Philadelphia, PA: F. A. Davis.

Walrafen, N., Brewer, M. K., & Mulvenon, C. (2012). Sadly caught up in the moment: An exploration of horizontal violence. *Nursing Economic$, 30*(1), 6–13.

Chapter 8: Critical Nursing Actions: Responding to Key Situations

American Nurses Association. (2003). *Scope and standards of nursing practice.* Silver Spring, MD: nursesbooks.org.

Caprio, A, J., Rollins, V. P., & Roberts, E. (2012). Health care professionals' perceptions and use of the Medical Orders for Scope of Treatment (MOST) Form in North Carolina nursing homes. *Journal of the American Medical Directors Association, 13*(2), 162–168.

Chan, B. L., Witt, R., Charrow, A. P., Magee, A., et al. (2007). Mirror therapy for phantom limb pain. *New England Journal of Medicine, 357*(21), 2206–2207.

DeSpelder, L. A., & Strickland, A. L. (2010). *The last dance: Encountering death and dying* (9th ed.). Boston, MA: McGraw-Hill.

Dillon, P. M. (2007). *Nursing health assessment: A critical thinking case studies approach* (2nd ed.). Philadelphia, PA: F. A. Davis.

End-of-Life Nursing Education Consortium (ELNEC) FACT SHEET. (2013). Retrieved from the American Association of Colleges of Nursing Web site: http://www.aacn.nche.edu/elnec/about/fact-sheet

Grbach, W. (2007). Teaching strategies: *Reformulating SBAR to "I-SBAR-R."* Retrieved from http://qsen.org/?s = I-SBAR-R

Hoyert, D. L., & Xu, J. (2012). Deaths: Preliminary data for 2011. *National Vital Statistics Reports, 61*(6).

Hsu, I., Saha, S., Korthuis, P. T., Sharp, V., Cohn, J., Moore, R. D., & Beach, M. C. (2012). Providing support to patients in emotional encounters: A new perspective on missed empathic opportunities. *Patient Education and Counseling, 88*(3), 436–442.

Joint Commission. (2013). *National patient safety goals.* Oakbrook Terrace, IL: Author. Retrieved from http://www.jointcommission.org/standards_information/npsgs.aspx

Joint Commission. (2013). Facts about the official list of "do not use" abbreviations. Oakbrook Terrace, IL: Author. Retrieved from http://www.jointcommission.org/standards_information/npsgs.aspx

Kalisch, B. J., McLaughlin, M., & Dabney, B. W. (2012). Patient perceptions of missed nursing care. *Joint Commission Journal on Quality & Patient Safety, 38*(4), 161–167.

Matzo, M. L. (2004). Palliative care: Prognostication and the chronically ill. *American Journal of Nursing, 104*(9), 40–49.

McHugh, M. E., Miller-Saultz, D., Wuhrman, E., & Kosharskyy, B. (2012). Interventional pain management in the palliative care patient. *International Journal of Palliative Nursing, 18*(9), 426–433.

McNamara, M. C., Harmon, D., & Saunders, J. (2012). Effect of education on knowledge, skills and attitudes around pain. *British Journal of Nursing, 21*(16), 958–964.

Moura, V. L., Faurot, K. R., Gaylord, S. A., Mann, J. D., Sill, M., Lynch, C., & Lee, M. Y. (2012). Mind-body interventions for treatment of phantom limb pain in persons with amputation. *American Journal of Physical Medicine & Rehabilitation, 91*, 701–714. doi: 10.1097/PHM.0b013e3182466034

Myers, M., & Eckes, E. J. (2012). A novel approach to pain management in persons with sickle cell disease. *Medsurg Nursing, 21*(5), 293-297.

Pucci, A. R. (2010). *Feel the way you want to feel . . . no matter what!* Bloomington, IN: iUniverse.

Ray, M. A. (2010). *Transcultural caring dynamics in nursing and health care.* Philadelphia, PA: F. A. Davis.

Reed, C. C., Beadle, R. D., Gerhardt, S. D., Kongable, G. L., & Stewart, R. M. (2011). Case discussion in blood glucose variability. *Journal of Neuroscience Nursing, 43*(2), 70–76.

SBAR Technique for Communication: A situational briefing model. (2011). Retrieved from Institute for Healthcare Improvement Web site: http://www.ihi.org/knowledge/Pages/Tools/SBARTechniqueforCommunicationASituational BriefingModel.aspx

Scherder, E. J. A., & Plooji, B. (2012). Assessment and management of pain, with particular emphasis on central neuropathic pain, in moderate to severe dementia. *Drugs & Aging, 29*(9), 701–706.

Stecher, J. (2008). "Allow natural death" vs. "Do not resuscitate": A kinder, gentler approach would benefit everyone. *American Journal of Nursing, 108*(7), 11.

Urgelles, J., Donohue, B., Wilks, C., Van Hasselt, V. B., & Azrin, N. H. (2012). A standardized method of preventing and managing emergencies within the context of evidence-based therapy implementation. *Behavior Modification, 36*, 558–579. doi: 10.1177/0145445512448192

U.S. Department of Health and Human Services, Centers for Disease Control and Prevention. (2008, June 11). *National Vital Statistics Reports Deaths: Preliminary data for 2006.* Retrieved from http://www.cdc.gov/nchs/products/pubs/pubd/nvsr/nvsr.htm#vol56

Vargas-Schaffer, G. (2010). Is the WHO analgesic ladder still valid? *Canadian Family Physician, 56*(6), 514–517.

Venneman, S., Narnor-Harris, P., Perish, M., & Hamilton, M. (2008). Allow natural death versus do not resuscitate: Three words that can change a life. *Journal of Medical Ethics, 34*(2), 2–6.

Whitcomb, J. J., & Ewing, N. (2012). A closing word: Do Not Resuscitate versus Allow Natural Death and should we change our approach? *Dimensions of Critical Care Nursing, 31*, 265–266. doi: 10.1097/DCC.0b013e318256e29d

Chapter 9: Ethics: Addressing Dilemmas in Professional Practice

American Nurses Association. (2004). *Foundations of nursing package.* Washington, DC: nursesbooks.org.

American Nurses Association. (2009). *Genetics/genomics nursing: Scope and standards of practice* (2nd ed.). Washington, DC: nursesbooks.org.

Ascension Health Care. (2007). *Healthcare ethics.* St. Louis, MO: Author.

Badzek, L., Turner, M., & Jenkins, J. (2008). Genomics and nursing practice: Advancing the nursing profession. *OJIN: The Online Journal of Issues in Nursing, 13*(1).

Berger, M. C., Seversen, A., & Chvatal, R. (1991). Ethical issues in nursing. *Western Journal of Nursing Research, 13*(4), 514–521.

Campbell, L. (2012). *A genomics primer* (2nd ed.). Denver, CO: Regis University.

Cherry, B., & Jacob, S. R. (2011). *Contemporary nursing: Issues, trends, and management* (5th ed.). St. Louis, MO: Mosby.

Cystic Fibrosis Foundation. (2013). *Frequently asked questions.* Bethesda, MD: Author. Retrieved from http://www.cff.org/AboutCF/Faqs/#What_is_the_life_expectancy_for_people_who_have_CF_(in_the_United_States)?

Gaffney, T. (2008). The need to go green. *Virginia Nurses Today, 16*(2), 11.

International Council of Nurses. (2012). *The ICN Code of Ethics for Nurses, revised.* Geneva, Switzerland: Author.

318

Jenkins, J. F., & Lea, D. H. (2005). *Nursing care in the genomic era: A case-based approach.* Sudbury, MA: Jones & Bartlett.

Laustsen, G. (2010). Greening in healthcare. *Nursing Management: The Journal of Excellence in Nursing Leadership, 41*(11), 26–31. doi: 10.1097/01.NUMA.0000389012.829989.5d

Laustsen, G. (2010). How green is your OR? *OR Nurse, 4*(3), 47–52.

Laustsen, G. R. (2005). *Promoting ecological behavior in nurses through action research* (doctoral dissertation). Denver, CO: University of Colorado Denver College of Nursing. UMI Order # AAI3168656.

Laustsen, G. R. (2007). Reduce—recycle—reuse: Guidelines for promoting perioperative waste management. *AORN Journal, 85*(4), 717–722, 724, 726–728.

McDonough, W., & Braungart, M. (2002). *Cradle to cradle: Remaking the way we make things.* New York, NY: North Point Press.

National Human Genome Research Institute. (2011). *A brief guide to genomics.* Retrieved from http://www.genome.gov/18016863

National Human Genome Research Institute. (2013). *Genetic discrimination and other laws.* Retrieved from http://www.genome.gov/10002077

National Human Genome Research Institute. (2009). *Genetic information nondiscrimination act of 2008.* Retrieved from http://www.genome.gov/10002328

Practice Greenhealth. (2012). *Sustainability benchmark report.* Reston, VA: Author.

Project C.U.R.E. (2013). *A remarkable history.* Retrieved from http://www.projectcure.org/about/history

Santos, E. M. M., Edwards, Q. T., Floria-Santos, M., Rogatto, S. R., Achatz, M. I. W., & MacDonald, D. J. (2013). Integration of genomics in cancer care. *Journal of Nursing Scholarship, 45*, 43–51. doi: 10.1111/j.1547-5069.2012.01465.x

U.S. Environmental Protection Agency. (2012). *Reduce, reuse, recycle.* Retrieved from http://www.epa.gov/wastes/conserve/rrr/

WebEcoist. (2008). *A brief history of the modern Green Movement in America.* Retrieved from http://webecoist.momtastic.com/2008/08/17/a-brief-history-of-the-modern-green-movement/

Chapter 10: Next Steps: Advancing in Your Career

Byrne, R. (2006). *The secret.* New York, NY: Atria.

Campbell, L. (2013). *Moving Mountains self care framework* (3rd ed.). Denver, CO: Moving Mountains (movingmountains-chs@hotmail.com).

Cooper, C. (2001). *The art of nursing: A practical introduction.* Philadelphia, PA: Saunders.

Covey, S., Merrill, A. R., & Merrill, R. R. (1994). *First things first: To live, to love, to learn, to leave a legacy.* New York, NY: Simon & Schuster.

DeBruyn, R. L. (2008). Seven motivators you can use all year long. *The Professor in the Classroom, 15*(3), 1–5.

Gladwell, M. (2002). *The tipping point: How little things can make a big difference.* New York, NY: Back Bay Books.

Hudacek, S. S. (2008). Dimensions of caring: A qualitative analysis of nurses' stories. *Journal of Nursing Education, 47*(3), 124–129.

Loehr, J., & Schwartz, T. (2005). *The power of full engagement.* New York, NY: The Free Press.

Lowney, C. (2003). *Heroic leadership.* Chicago, IL: Loyola Press.

Lowney, C. (2009). *Heroic living.* Chicago, IL: Loyola Press.

Meehan, T. C. (2003). Careful nursing: A model for contemporary nursing practice. *Journal of Advanced Nursing 44*(1), 99–107.

Pender, N. J., Murdaugh, C., & Parsons, M. A. (2010). *Health promotion in nursing practice* (6th ed.). Upper Saddle River, NJ: Prentice-Hall Health.

Putre, L. (2013). A clash of ages: Are you bridging the generation gap in your medical and nursing staff? *Hospitals and Health Networks, 87*(3), 40–44.

Ruiz, D. M. (1997). *The four agreements: A practical guide to personal freedom.* Carlsbad, CA: Hay House.

Ryan, L. (2013). Your personal brand is more than just your job. *Bloomberg Businessweek.* New York, NY: Bloomberg LP. Retrieved from http://www.businessweek.com/articles/2013-02-19/your-personal-brand-is-more-than-just-your-job

ILLUSTRATION CREDIT LIST

Figure 1–1 is based on Benner, P. (2001). *From novice to expert: Excellence and power in clinical nursing practice* (commemorative ed.). Upper Saddle River, NJ: Prentice Hall.

Figures 3–2, 3–3, 3–4, 3–5, 8–1, and 8–2 are from Dillon, P. M. (2007). *Nursing health assessment: A critical thinking, case studies approach* (2nd ed.). Philadelphia, PA: F. A. Davis.

Figures 5–1, 5–2, 5–3, 5–7, 5–8, 5–9, 5–10, 5–11, 5–12, and 5–14 are from Wilkinson, J.M., & Van Leuven, K. (2008). *Fundamentals of nursing.* Philadelphia, PA: F. A. Davis.

Figures 5–4, 5–5, 5–6, 5–13, and 5–15 are from Rhoads, J. and Meeker, B. J. (2008). *Davis's guide to clinical nursing skills.* Philadelphia, PA: F. A. Davis.

Figure 7–3 was created by Wendeline J. Grbach, MSN, RN CCRN, CLNC; reprinted with permission.

Figure 8–3 is adapted from the World Health Organization's pain ladder, retrieved from http://www.who.int

Figure 10–1 is adapted from Covey, S. R., Merrill, A. R., Merrill, R. R. (1994). *First things first.* New York, NY: Simon & Schuster, p. 37.

Index

Note: Page numbers followed by "b," "f," and "t" indicate boxes, figures, and tables, respectively.